THE POWER & PAIN
OF NURSING

Copyright © 2021 Beth Cavenaugh
All rights reserved. No part of this publication may be reproduced, distributed, or transmitted in any form or by any means, including photocopying, recording, or other electronic or mechanical methods, without the prior written permission of the publisher, except in the case of brief quotations embodied in critical reviews and certain other noncommercial uses permitted by copyright law. For permission requests, write to the publisher, addressed "Attention: Permissions Coordinator," at the address below.

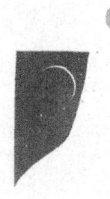

Sun and Moon Press
moonandsunpress@gmail.com

Cover and illustrations by Julia Cone

ISBN: 978-1-7336909-2-8 (print)
ISBN: 978-1-7336909-3-5 (ebook)

Ordering Information:
Special discounts are available on quantity purchases by corporations, associations, and others. For details, contact moonandsunpress@gmail.com

This book is dedicated to all front-line workers during the pandemic. This includes anyone who worked in *any* health care setting in 2020 (and 2021). *Thank you* feels inadequate. *I love you* feels awkward. *I am in awe* feels right.

Table of Contents

Introduction	9
Day 1 – Compassion: The Call to Alleviate Suffering	13
Day 2 – Locating Breath	17
Day 3 – Dear God and Jesus and Buddha and Allah	21
Day 4 – A Mango and Some Chocolate	25
Day 5 – Ponder, Palpate, Percuss	29
Day 6 – Gratitude Festival	31
Day 7 – Bleary-Eyed, Sleepless, Saliva-Less	35
Day 8 – You Can Do It All, but Why?	39
Day 9 – You Are Insignificant and Significant	43
Day 10 – The Ferocious Love of Family	47
Day 11 – Advocating for Your Patients	51
Day 12 – Just One Intentional Minute	55
Day 13 – Pie	59
Day 14 – Super-Friggin Hero	63
Day 15 – No No No No No	67
Day 16 – A Soft, Fluffy, Edgy Nurse	71

Day 17 – Marshmallows and Peanut Butter	75
Day 18 – *How* Care Is Delivered	79
Day 19 – Dirty Children	83
Day 20 – Sparkles in the Carpet	85
Day 21 – Hoist, Hustle, Hurdle	87
Day 22 – Healing Touch	91
Day 23 – Simple Gestures Lead to the Sacred	93
Day 24 – Divine Flow	95
Day 25 – Am I Dying?	99
Day 26 – A Holy Shift	103
Day 27 – Get the Fluffy Tissues	109
Day 28 – Secondhand Trauma	113
Day 29 – A Soft Front and a Strong Back	117
Day 30 – Too Much Fight or Flight	121
Conclusion – A Love Letter to Nurses	123
Bibliography	127
Acknowledgements	131

THE POWER & PAIN OF NURSING

SELF-CARE PRACTICES TO PROTECT & REPLENISH COMPASSION

Beth Cavenaugh RN, BSN, CHPN with
Dominic O. Vachon MDiv, PhD
MJ Murray Vachon LCSW, LMFT

Introduction

My cousin MJ called me up week three of the pandemic to see if I was interested in collaborating on a mental health program for health care professionals. As a hospice nurse, a mother of three kids, and a human, I felt a little unglued myself. I said, "Um, h*ll yes." So, four professionals got together via Zoom, and we realized we had the perfect storm. I have boots-on-the-ground clinical nursing experience, MJ Murray Vachon, LCSW, LMFT, has spent her life as a therapist, Colleen Sweeney, RN, CSP, has spent years working with hospital systems to develop more empathy toward patients, and Dominic Vachon MDiv, PhD, professor at University of Notre Dame and Director of the Hillebrand Center for Compassionate Care in Medicine has spent the last 26 years in clinical practice while researching, writing, and teaching about the science of compassion in medicine. We created a program of urgent self-care for health care professionals called the Heroes' Huddle.

In those months of writing and collaborating to develop critical science-based tools for clinicians, I had many "Aha!" moments. I realized I had spent the last 24 years of my own nursing career learning how to take care of myself so I would not be ruined by the intensity of clinical work. I meditated, I went on retreats, I read, I napped, I underfunctioned at home, I did body scans and guided meditations, I took yoga classes, I walked among the trees, I prayed to the Earth and God and Jesus and Buddha and anyone else who would listen, and I paid for therapists, energy healers, and acupuncturists. I was constantly looking for tools that would renew my spirit from the intensity of nursing and the profound suffering of my patients. I wanted to be emotionally supportive and available to my patients *and* still have something left for my husband, my kids, and myself.

Dominic's research on the science of compassion helped me to understand why I had worked so hard on my inner life over the last 24 years, and Colleen's wisdom in patient care was vital to deepening my understanding of empathy fatigue, which I had experienced over the course of my career. MJ's therapeutic skills and experience with breathwork, rumination, and the mind-body connection would have been invaluable practices for me 24 years ago. Now I have the understanding, the research, and the words to describe what I have been striving for in my nursing practice: empathy, compassion, composure, emotional connection, and stillness. The good news is that these characteristics can be learned and are intimately tied to keeping you satisfied and productive throughout your career in health care.

INTRODUCTION

I wrote this book because the science of compassion shows that developing the ability to genuinely care for the people you serve improves patient satisfaction and health care outcomes while protecting the clinician from burnout (Vachon, 2020). As soon as nurses start their clinicals in school, they can (and should) begin to train their mind, body, and soul for difficult work. Your career can be an ongoing journey of self-care, self-awareness, self-help, self-love, self-compassion, and self-renewal (rather than exhaustion and depletion). If I had known about the science of compassion long ago, my life would have been much easier. In short, I am hoping to save you some time and money while improving patient outcomes.

This guidebook aims to inspire and encourage as you develop practices to maintain your compassion conditioning. It includes simple and effective science-based tools to take care of yourself, so that you can compassionately take care of your patients, your people, and most importantly, yourself. The daily practices include action, mindfulness, meditation, or embodiment exercises to facilitate your return to center. The most important practice, however, is being compassionate with yourself. Open this book in whatever way feels right to you. Most practices will benefit from a journal, some time, and some space. Perhaps pick this book up when you are feeling particularly burned out and crispy or choose a practice that calls to you. Maybe carve out a one-month period to work through 30 days before getting ready for work — with the absolute condition that you will not be hard on yourself if you miss a day. Take what inspires, develop your own practices, and leave what does not resonate.

When medical care is delivered in a compassionate and composed way, patients feel safe and trust the clinician. When care is evident and trust has been established, the patient will disclose more and will likely follow through with treatment plans, making health care outcomes better overall (Vachon, 2020). When clinicians can access their compassion and kindness while delivering medical care, they will experience more equanimity and satisfaction in their work and less burnout overall. Everyone wins.

If you want to stay grounded, be resilient, and maintain a compassionate mindset in health care (and your home life), you simply must have self-care and mental wellness practices woven into, throughout, over, and under your life. This book aims to be your scaffolding. It will support you through the intensity of this work.

Thank you for the beautiful work that you do.

Beth Cavenaugh RN, BSN, CHPN

Day 1

Compassion: The Call to Alleviate Suffering

When Dr. Dominic Vachon said to me, "Compassion is when clinicians notice suffering and are moved to do all they can within their competency and role to alleviate that suffering," I wanted to weep. I thought, "Oh my God, nurses should get paid millions of dollars."

I look back on my near-quarter century of nursing and am struck by all that I did with such vehemence to eliminate my patients' suffering. I had one patient who suddenly went into respiratory distress. In response, I ran to the Pyxis to get meds to alleviate their air hunger, called on a volunteer to sit with the patient, asked my co-worker to watch out for my other patients, and summoned the doctor, knowing I would need a more comprehensive medical approach for this respiratory event. All of that took about 15 minutes. Both the patient and I were sweating by the end of the crisis, but finally, he could breathe easier. I could breathe easier too.

Nurses are always giving their patients this level of urgent love. Most people have no idea how hard we are sweating in our cotton-polyester blend scrubs.

Every nurse is dedicated and committed to the call to alleviate suffering. This is your *why*. Not many people choose this *why* for a profession. There should be a party for you every day, a party with streamers, balloons, and sexy people jumping out of cakes.

Self-Care Practice

A genuine desire to alleviate a patient's suffering is a requirement for being a nurse. Sometimes, though, this call to alleviate suffering can transform into fatigue and overwhelm. Research on the science of compassion shows that "when a clinician can stay connected to their genuine desire to care for their patients, it can improve patient outcomes and buffer burnout" (Vachon, 2020). For the next 20 minutes, you will journal about what drives you as a nurse.

Sit in a chair and ground yourself by moving your awareness to your feet. Follow your breath until you feel anchored in the present. Now call to mind a recent patient or family you felt connected to, and for a few minutes, run a movie in your mind remembering this experience with as much detail as possible. What did you do to build trust? How did you offer information? What actions did you take to provide treatment in a caring and comforting way?

After reflecting, consider how the outcomes changed because of your caring, competence, and compassion. Now is not the time to minimize or downplay your powerful role. Write about your realizations.

Now, reflect specifically on your *why*.

Why did you become a nurse? Is there any overlap to your story? How does it feel when you alleviate the physical, emotional, or spiritual suffering of your patients? What are the factors involved in accomplishing these? Be overwhelmed with what you love about nursing or the impact you can make on someone's life. Steep in it, dwell on it, and roll around in it.

As the weeks go on, come back to this page in your journal for ongoing inspiration.

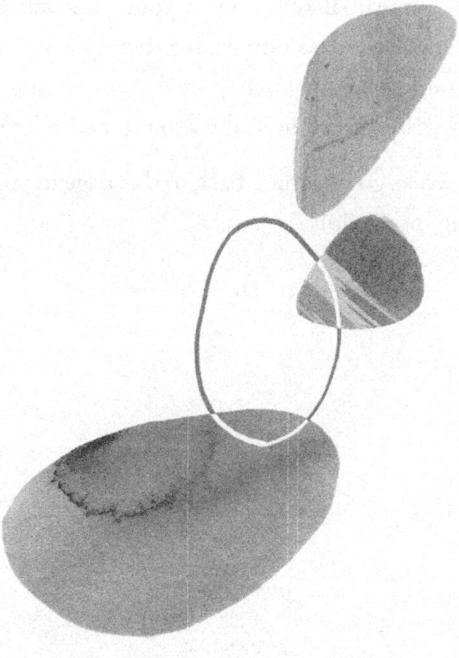

Day 2

Locating Breath

We take breath for granted until it is difficult to breathe.

No profession knows and fights for the ability to breathe more than yours. You encourage patients to use their incentive spirometers, you administer oxygen, morphine, inhalers, and nebulizers, and you vigilantly listen for changing breath sounds. When you perform CPR, you wait with your own suspended breath for the inhale. When the inhale comes, you exhale, and you know deep in your alveoli that this is a noble cause — the fight for your patient's breath.

Self-Care Practice

You may find yourself holding your own breath when one of your patients is angry, vomiting, in pain, in respiratory distress, or dying.[1] Intentional breathwork can be a form of

---

[1] According to Stephen Porges' research on the science of compassion, when one is feeling empathy toward another's suffering, it may trigger a fight-or-flight response. Compassion, however, "respects the individual's capacity to experience their own pain ... which contributes to the healing process" (Porges, 2021, p. 70).

mindfulness that helps you redirect your attention to focus on one simple thing rather than your mind's constant chatter. Breathwork can also activate your parasympathetic nervous system, which can counter your body's fight-or-flight response (Porges, 2017).[2]

Today, you will spend some time connecting with your breath and learning a few techniques to draw upon during stressful moments. For instance, I often find myself holding my breath when I am managing my patient's pain. I do not think about my breath until I leave the room and start breathing again.

Find a quiet room and a comfortable seat. Set your timer for 15 minutes. Start by noticing. Where can you connect most easily with your breath? Is it at the nose, the chest, or the abdomen?

Slow Breathing Techniques[3]

Focus on your diaphragm, and feel the inhale expand your diaphragm, allowing you to fill up your lungs. Pause. As you exhale, focus on the diaphragm contracting as you expel the stale air from the bases of your lungs. Repeat for five minutes.

---

2   "Polyvagal theory explains how the rituals associated with contemplative practices (e.g., breathing, meditation) trigger physiological states that calm neural defense systems and promote feelings of safety that may lead to expressing and feeling compassion" (Porges, 2017, p 192).

3   This article reviewed the literature and found "evidence of increased psychophysiological flexibility linking parasympathetic activity, CNS activities related to emotional control, and psychological well-being in healthy subjects during slow breathing (6 breaths/min)" (Zaccaro, et al., 2018).

Square Breathing

Try slowly inhaling as you count to five. Hold for five more counts. Slowly exhale as you count to five again. Hold for five. Repeat for the next five minutes (Gotter & Weatherspoon, 2020).

Extending Your Exhale

Now, try inhaling slowly for the count of four, hold for seven, and exhale slowly for eight. A longer exhale increases the amount of CO_2 in your blood, which activates the parasympathetic nervous system. When you are breathing in either duration, concentrate on your breathing in the lower part of your lungs, expanding your belly as you breathe. Continue this breathwork for five minutes (Seppälä et al., 2020).

As you become more connected to your body and how you are responding to stress, you can quickly draw upon any of these simple breathing exercises when needed. Even 20 seconds of intentional breathing can help you center at any point in your day.

Day 3

Dear God and Jesus and Buddha and Allah

Courage is being afraid but showing up anyway. Working in health care, you have no choice. You must show up.

I had a hospice patient who had a sudden terminal event — his tumor likely invaded the carotid artery. He began to bleed out. I was terrified. I grabbed two co-workers, and I ran back and forth to the Pyxis to increase his meds for sedation, agitation, and pain management. I left the room three times to get more meds. The family was outside the room on a couch, watching me pretend like everything was OK. They knew he was dying but did not want to be in the room with him.

Every time I went back into the room, I waved to the family and silently said a little prayer: "Dear God, Jesus, Buddha, Allah, all the saints, and anyone else who will listen — help me, help me, help me!" I would then tell myself to just get in there and face my fears. It was a horrendous scene. Blood was everywhere.

We got him comfortable and helped make his death as beautiful and peaceful as possible with our presence and sufficient medications minimizing his discomfort. I do not cry during my shifts, but I sobbed that day right over the patient after he died.

My co-workers and I had a few minutes of pause, prayer, and silence. I blew my nose and pulled it together so I could gently tell the family he had died.

Self-Care Practice

According to recent research on fear and emotional regulation, trying to suppress our fears may intensify them or have devastating physical or emotional side effects. When we get clear about what we are afraid of — and there is a lot to fear in health care — we can deal with our fears more effectively (Dillard et al., 2018). I personally have had to deal with many fears while working: fear of my own mortality, fear of sputum, fear of vomit, fear of coronavirus, and the list goes on.[4]

The following exercise is called SIFTing the mind adapted from Dan Siegel. It is a great practice for clinicians, as we tend to numb ourselves to get through our intense shifts (Sie-

---

4   Dillard, Yang, and Li (2018) write that "fear has also been associated with diminished cardiovascular health, decreased immune functioning, and degraded psychological well-being."

gel, 2015).[5,6] This exercise is a process of naming what you are thinking and feeling so that you can calm your body and mind. You can then access the clarity needed to move forward. This is a practice to cultivate when you are not at work, but the more you do it, the more powerful it will be in any situation, even during an intense shift.

Find a quiet place and sit. Feel your feet contacting the ground and take seven breaths. Bring yourself into the present moment.

Close your eyes, if you are comfortable doing so, and turn your attention inward.

Notice what is going on inside of you.

Notice the *sensations* in your body (such as tension, knotted stomach, peace, clamped jaw, headache, or calm).

Take some more intentional breaths.

Notice if any *images* come into your mind. (These images could feel random or not: a beach, an airplane crashing, a church, streamers, your supervisor, a slice of pizza, etc.)

Take some intentional breaths.

Notice what you are *feeling* (sadness, relief, dread, doom, fear, pride, excitement, adrenaline, etc.).

---

5   Yes, this exercise is from a book about the teenage brain. I do not know about you, but I grew up shoving my emotions under the carpet and began to access the power of my emotions later in adulthood. I personally find this exercise helpful.

6   This exercise was adapted by MJ Murray Vachon from Dan Siegel's book, *The Whole-Brain Child: 12 Revolutionary Strategies to Nurture Your Child's Developing Mind*.

Pause.

Notice your *thoughts*. (Holy shizzle, I am so tired. I must go home. I have to pee. I need help. That went better than expected.)

You have just sifted through your inner world, your world that is so easy to ignore with all the outside demands placed on you.

Make note of what sensations, images, feelings, and thoughts you noticed.

Some of what you noticed may need attention, such as sleep, food, a conversation with your supervisor, or a celebration for everything you did today.

Some of it may just need to be noticed.

This quick exercise can help guide you in how best to take care of yourself after a long day of caring for others.

Day 4

A Mango and Some Chocolate

One of the most difficult aspects of working in health care is that intensity always surrounds you. You tend to patients with horrific burns or a shattered pelvis from a fall, you feel the inequities or the misfortune of some, and you wander into a room heavy with grief or trauma. There is no screaming or backing away. You walk calmly into it. After 12 hours, you stroll to your car, stop at the grocery store, and select a mango as if you had not just been covered with blood or seen a beautiful child's last breath. You pay for your perfectly ripe mango, and let us be honest, some chocolate. You go home, shower, and empty the dishwasher as if nothing big happened over the course of the day.

Self-Care Practice

For me, it was always easier to tend to the dishes than to my emotions, my sadness, and my "holy sh*t" moments. But as you know, these emotions will show up at some point — and usually when you least expect it. These emotions may insidiously creep into your cells and become insomnia, anxiety, or depression. The science of compassion reveals that clinicians who take time to reflect and process their emotions do better in the long run than clinicians who suppress or deny the emotional cost of this difficult work (Vachon, 2020). Today, you are going to brainstorm creative practices to physically process and release the emotional intensity of your work.

To help regulate our emotions as mature humans, we must practice moving from reaction to reflection. As we thoughtfully process our emotions, we can free our body *and* our mind. Our body will be able to metabolize the feeling in a healthy way rather than warehousing it, and our mind will be capable of sorting and decision making. (MJ Murray Vachon, personal communication, April 2020).

Spend some time reflecting on a recent shift. Are there any reactions or intense feelings that begin to percolate? Name and acknowledge these feelings. ("Oh, there you are, anger. Oh, heavy sadness again — hi, honey.")

Where do these emotions land in your body? Place a hand here and gently breathe into this space for 90 seconds. You will notice a dissipation of the tension there. You are moving from a reactive mind to a wise mind — a mind that can integrate rational and emotional information. As your body calms, listen to what your body wants to do next. Typically, the body will guide you to a simple solution, such as a taking a walk, writing in your journal, or connecting with a friend.

If you are still having a lot of emotions and feel as though your body needs a little bit more, you can choose one of these activities to do with all your might. Pay attention to ensure that you are not aggravating the emotions and building the story into something much larger than it is.[7] Here are some ideas:

- Dance out your depressed mood.
- Flambe your f**k you-feelings.
- Jog out your judgment.
- Artistically unleash your annoyance.
- Bake away your bitterness.
- Sleep off your sadness.
- Garden out your grief.
- Kickbox your crustiness to the curb.

The purpose of this exercise is to honor your emotions and give them the time and space to integrate, soften, and then wisely inform your next steps.

---

7   When I am angry at someone, I like to listen to Lily Allen's "F**k You" song repeatedly. Though very satisfying, it does not help me to move forward. It simply builds the story while feeding the anger and self-righteousness. So, pay attention — are you calming the emotions or fueling them?

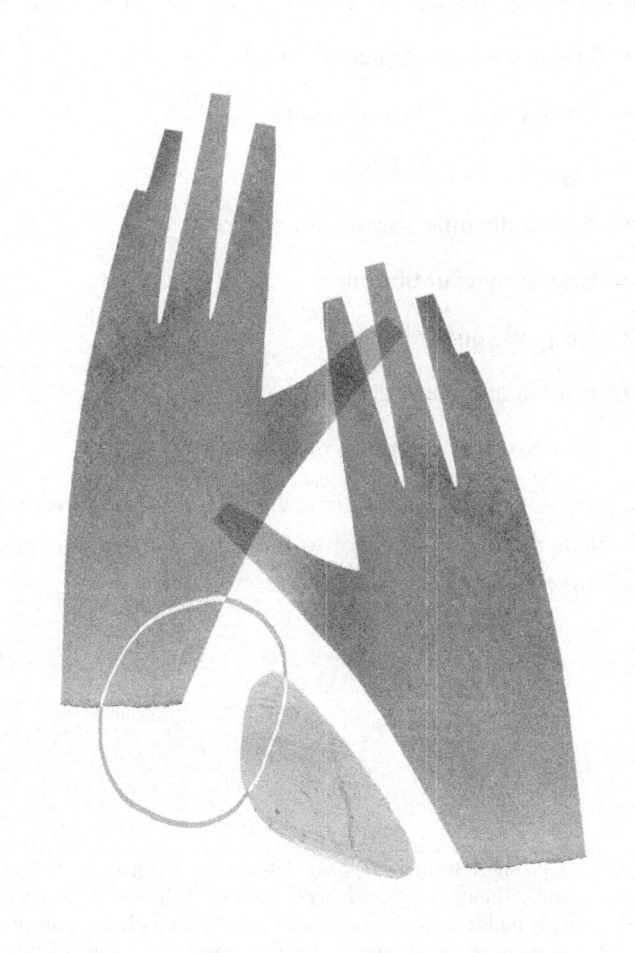

Day 5

Ponder, Palpate, Percuss

I still remember my postpartum nurse 17 years after giving birth to my daughter. Shortly after Lillijane burst into the world with a kick*ss Apgar and a lusty cry, I began to hemorrhage. My nurse sprang into action. She pounced on my abdomen and "massaged" my aching fundus like bread dough. It hurt. So bad. I cannot recall what this nurse looked like, but I do remember her swift response, her competence, and her incredibly strong hands. I love this nameless, faceless nurse with every fiber of my being, even a decade and a half later.

Self-Care Practice

The practice of appreciating your hands can connect you with the physical and healing work that you do repeatedly under difficult circumstances.

For today's practice, appreciate the power of your healing hands.

Grab some lotion and take a seat. Thoughtfully massage your

hands with lotion while considering your dry, cracked, and overworked hands. They rarely get a break. They do *everything*. They hang blood, they titrate medications, and they perform meticulous wound care and rapid clinical procedures. They ponder, palpate, and percuss. They assess, they communicate, they hold, and they bless. And they get sanitized over and over and over again.

Bless your dry, raw (but still perfect) hands. Rub them together and feel the warmth and energy build up between them. These blessed hands are healing our world one patient at a time.

Marvel at your hands, appreciate them, and let them hold and heal you for a change.

Day 6

Gratitude Festival

Some days I feel a little bit grumpy about nursing in general. It may be my age and hormonal situation, but I can easily slide into the negative. Why do we have to run from patient to patient? Why do I not get hazard pay for every shift? Why is being understaffed the norm? *Bitch bitch, moan moan.* ... Although these are legitimate concerns and not issues to be swept under the carpet, this negativity can easily spiral and usually does nothing for my mood or staff morale.

Most humans tend toward the negative. Positivity is a decision one must actively make and practice.[8] Gratitude can have an overwhelmingly positive effect on your outlook. It is associated with decreased stress, increased altruism, and improved social relationships (Emmons & Mishra, 2011). Today's practice is not meant to ignore your legitimate concerns about the

---

8 My cousin MJ and I have long talks. She is brilliant, and I rely on her to help me get back on track. Some days I have to work harder than others at being positive. She reminds me that we must *choose* positivity.

health care system or your profession, but it may help you to find some relief and clarity. Gratitude is like throwing ice water on your perspective — in a good way.

Self-Care Practice

Today, we will spend some time practicing a co-worker gratitude festival. Health care is a collaborative, team-centered, and synergistic approach to optimizing the wellness of your patient. Compassion science research has found that collegial support in an organization is one of the major ways to keep morale up and buffer burnout (Vachon, 2020).

Reflecting on your last few shifts, when did you need:

- Four hands to hoist the patient from the chair to the bed?
- A strong back to gently roll and hold a patient while you dressed a wound?
- Information from the CNA who always knows more than they say they do?
- The night shift nurse to follow up on a task you did not complete?
- The day shift nurse to follow up and clarify the discharge orders?
- A nurse who could talk you through a difficult catheter placement while lighting your way?
- A social work savior who would find resources for your homeless patient?
- A physician to quickly give you whatever orders you want?

- A transparent colleague who would tell you to put some deodorant on?

- A prayer of support from the chaplain because some days you need it?

- Your manager to run interference with a distressed family member?

Contemplate your teammates and their vital role in making you look like an excellent nurse. Write down some instances, and on your next shift, thank your co-workers for a specific something they did. Intentional gratitude for our colleagues can shake us out of our negative patterns and benefit staff morale while softening our way in the world.[9]

---

9 Gratitude is a virtue that we must cultivate. Other benefits from Mishra and Emmons' (2011) research shows gratitude is associated with a more forgiving outlook, spiritual transcendence, less envy, less materialism, improved confidence, and increased motivation of social behavior. Hmmm. Seems like gratitude is the antidote to everything bad — and it is free.

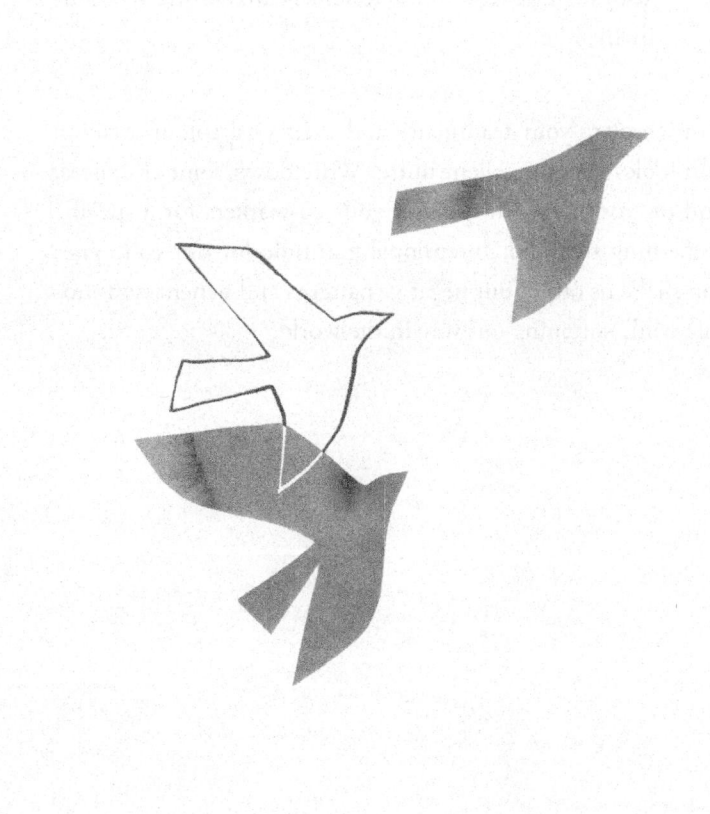

Day 7

Bleary-Eyed, Sleepless, Saliva-Less

Every clinician is an educator. You are constantly teaching patients about their health, their body, their discharge instructions, their pain medications, their knee exercises, their new diet, their insulin injections, and their wound care. You answer questions all day, every day.

You also teach your colleagues — you scrape together your last morsels of patience at the end of your shift and teach your colleagues new skills and protocols. You pivot and practice with new equipment and supplies; the old impart their pearls of wisdom, and the young teach the old about social media. When nurses are afraid to ask questions, insulted if they do not know something, or not given ample time or instruction to learn a new process, these are signs of a dangerous unit. When you openly acknowledge and cultivate your unit as an educational environment, it can contribute to a culture of safety, patience, humility, and respect between colleagues.

Jean Watson, nurse theorist and expert in the science of caring, finds that engaging in teaching and learning are major parts of the healing process both for the patient and nurse (Watson, 2008). I love this — teaching and learning can aid in our healing.

About a decade ago, I was asked to give a presentation to hospice volunteers — the next day. Their original presenter was sick, and I was the fifth person they asked. I readily agreed because teaching was something I had always wanted to pursue. That said, I have a bizarre fear of public speaking that goes back to the '90s.

I worked feverishly on this hospice presentation and consequently worked myself into an anxious frenzy. I had no reason to be afraid of hospice volunteers because they are the kindest humans on the planet. The next day, bleary-eyed, sleepless, and saliva-less, I delivered the presentation with the flat cadence of a recently anesthetized dental patient. I completed the talk, walked to my car, and had a strange physiological episode where I shook uncontrollably for five minutes.

Strangely, I wanted to teach more even though the feedback responses said, "Presentation was monotone," and "She was so nervous that it distracted from the content." I suddenly felt so passionate about teaching these kind-eyed volunteers about hospice. This started my mission to inform, educate, and write about end-of-life matters.

Self-Care Practice

For today's practice, you are going to play with possibilities. You do not need to do or commit to anything at all.

Turn on some music, get comfortable, and relax a bit. Let your mind wander as you consider being in the role of a student or a teacher. Do you have any areas of study you would like to learn about? Would you like to teach about something someday? It can be as simple as watching a port-a-cath access video or as lofty as directing a documentary about cancer patients. It does not have to be about nursing. It can be the inspiration to take a Thai cooking class or get certified to teach yoga. All areas of passion inform our nursing practice and fuel our hearts as humans, which fuel our hearts as nurses.

Sometimes we get a nudge. Sometimes we get hit over the head with an idea. Whatever form your desire to teach or learn takes, honor it, and give it some room to take shape. My book about end-of-life care was inspired by this thought: I want to either quit nursing and work in a pie shop or start a podcast about death and dying. I let these thoughts simmer, morph, and stretch. I took some time off nursing in between. Two years later, I published a bedside hospice guidebook. I never made one pie.

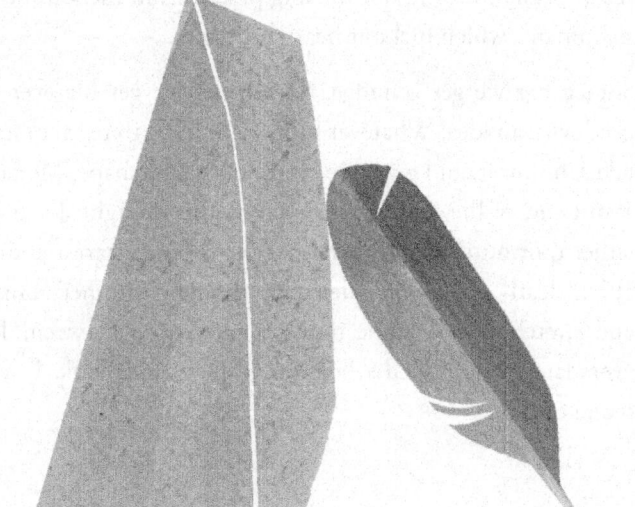

Day 8

You Can Do It All, but Why?

Although we have one specific job description, most days we do everything. In just one shift, you may be a housekeeper, chef, bouncer, family therapist, chaplain, and the departments of social work, security, and safety. As a nurse, I have taken care of my patients while conducting end-of-life ceremonies, leading heated family conferences, shoveling snow, emptying wastebaskets, scrambling eggs, and coordinating one wedding. Well, I oversaw the patient's 30 liters of oxygen before, during, and after their wedding, so I felt like an integral part of the ceremony.

Some days you may not feel equipped for the all-encompassing nature of this work, but remember that you *are*. You are a parent, a sibling, a friend, a partner, and a child. You have been playing multiple roles for years. Evolutionary biologists have confirmed that humans have incredible systems designed to respond to the pain and suffering of others. We rely on our clinical training to respond compassionately to our patients, but we can also rely on our experiences as daughters, sons, parents, and fellow human beings (Goetz et al., 2010; Vachon, 2020).

Self-Care Practice

Of course you can do it all, but that does not mean you should do it all. Healthy unit cultures have a built-in norm that everyone knows they can reach out to other team members to help when patients are particularly distressed or demanding, and I will add, at any time (Vachon, 2020).

I often forget that health care is better if it is collaborative. Nurses are bedside witnesses and critical to initiating this collaboration. The chaplain will never just saunter into a patient's room because of existential distress. It is our job to let them know Room 22 is struggling with relationships, grief, and spiritual pain. When patients or family members discuss their emotional or financial distress, I will ask the social worker to follow up with them. And CNAs are the tender hearts who reposition, clean up, and bathe patients when we ask them to.

When my patient casually mentioned her emotional distress over dying, I tried to help her process this, and after an awkward 10-minute conversation, I walked over to the doctor, social worker, and chaplain to ask for help. Over the course of the day, they were able to help this patient begin to process the physical reality of her disease, her emotional anguish, and her spiritual suffering — they had the skills necessary to navigate this emotional conversation. I thank my lucky stars every day I am part of a team.

Today, I want you to write a list of all the people you can call on to help you while you are working. The doctor, the chaplain, the social worker, the RT, the PT, the nutritionists, the nurses, the CNAs, or the manager.

Part of our job is to communicate with and delegate to these brilliant, skilled professionals when we are lost, confused, overwhelmed, underwhelmed, or have veered waaaaaay out of our lane. Thank goodness for the team approach.

Day 9

You Are Insignificant and Significant

Sometimes your role as a nurse can feel insignificant in terms of a patient's life circumstances. There are so many factors that are beyond your control that will affect your patient's health and healing: their biology, biochemistry, DNA, liver, kidneys, neural chemistry, blessings, misfortunes, optimism, negativity, financial security, poverty, the system, Medicare, Medicaid, spiritual strength, a difficult childhood, their home, supportive friends, or estranged families.

The good news is you have the opportunity to do what you can during your 12-hour shift, and that is significant.

One shift, I admitted a patient who was homeless, unresponsive, and actively dying from pancreatic cancer. His chart showed no family contacts, just the number of a homeless shelter. Our team flew into action. The social worker called the shelter, and two supportive staff members from the shelter adjusted their schedules so they could be with him in his final hours. The physician and I adjusted his medications to soften his labored breathing. The CNA tenderly bathed him and dressed him in a clean t-shirt and sweatpants.

The shelter workers arrived and sat near his bedside as he was dying, telling stories about the patient's quiet demeanor and his love for his morning coffee. They offered him coffee on a swab and stayed with him as he breathed his last breaths. I did not know how or why this patient was homeless, why he was estranged from his family, or why he had the misfortune of pancreatic cancer, but I do know that he died clean, blessed, comfortable, and surrounded by people who cared about him.

Once I was able to let go of what I absolutely could not control, I found some relief and was able to focus on what I could control.

Self-Care Practice

Compassion does not ignore suffering — it strengthens one's resolve to respond to the patient's suffering and provides consequential satisfaction and fulfillment for the clinician (Vachon, 2020).

This 20-minute practice can help you to recharge after an intense shift and give you space to distinguish between what you can and cannot change.

Take off your shoes and go outside. Feel the ground under your feet. Take some breaths and connect with the earth's energy below you. Imagine letting go of any energy that is not serving you at this moment. Let go of the worry and exhaustion you feel from the patients you encounter daily: the small child who is dying from cancer, your frequent flyer patients who return because they have no access to resources, or your patient's sucky life circumstances. Let it all go into the earth to be absorbed and neutralized — the earth can handle it.

Rest for a minute. These patient stories will help to shape and build your compassionate self.

Bless and thank the patients who came to mind.

Now, pull some of this powerful earth energy into your body. Imagine it flowing into your bones and your cells, filling you up with power and light. Imagine it circling in and out of your body and all around you. Take some deep breaths. Feel the new vibration and lightness in your body.[10]

There is so much we cannot control about our patient's life circumstances, and yet, we can still have a profound and significant impact during our 12-hour shift. This embodiment practice can serve as a visual and physical reminder of releasing and letting go of that which you cannot control.

---

10 My energetic awareness as a Reiki practitioner has only enhanced my practice as a nurse. When we allow ourselves to play with the subtleties of our energies and that which we cannot see, we can tap into our human spirit. We often talk about a patient's spirit, fight, or resolve. You can feel it in the room and watch with awe as they heal. This nuanced awareness may help you to see your patients with more clarity.

Day 10

The Ferocious Love of Family

Every mother, father, son, daughter, and partner has written a catastrophic ending when they hear their loved one is in the hospital. They are terrified of what the news could mean — the heart attack, the high fever, or the broken hip. They run into the hospital, and the only person they care about is their loved one. They want to know now what may take hours or days to diagnose or treat. They may hover around the nurses' station as they wait for test results. They will Google possible endings to the story and pace outside the staff lounge while panicked and drained. Your one patient becomes multiple patients (and insurance does not pay for supportive family members).

Anyone in health care knows that family is *always* a significant part of your shift: the phone calls, the tears, the grieving, the questions, the education, the sisters, the explanations, the aunties, and the adult children who are always physicians.

You *know* you would be the same powerful, relentless advocate, and because you are a nurse, you may be slightly more persistent and possibly intimidating. I took our cat Petunia to the vet hospital, and though I do not know the first thing about animal care, I offered many nursing suggestions from medications to supportive care at home. It is safe to say I was annoying.

Self-Care Practice

Nursing requires an inordinate amount of kindness. Your families are stressed, in crisis, grieving, scared, and often not in their right mind. I have been yelled at, blamed, interrupted, interrogated, and doubted. Our job is to not take this personally but to know in our hearts that their hearts are hurting, breaking, or exhausted. Contemplative practices, such as loving-kindness meditation, centering prayer, yoga, and mindfulness, can all help to increase your altruistic desire and your empathy toward strangers (Vachon, 2020; Dagar et al., 2020).

For today's practice, do a simple and gentle yoga practice. Because children and animals will find you, this may be a good practice to do in the main center of the house; let them join you. You are not sneaking time away from your family — you are modeling proper self-care.

Stand still, with your arms at your sides and breathe. Yoga is the union of mind, body, and spirit. It can serve as a meditation and centering practice.

Forward Fold

Stand straight with your arms hanging gently at your sides. Take an inhale and raise your hands up over your head. On the exhale, slowly swan dive forward, bringing your hands toward the ground. Let your head hang. You can bend your legs as much as you need or straighten the legs if that feels better. The goal is to feel good. Stretch out your spine and lower back. Let the blood flow to your head. With each exhale, release a little more.

Tabletop

From the forward fold position, pace your hands on the ground so they line up with your shoulders. Then place your knees on the ground so your knees line up with your hips. From tabletop position, play with any position that allows your spine and sides to stretch and release.

Inhale as you gently drop your abdomen toward the earth for cow pose, and exhale as you extend your back into cat pose, stretching along your spine. You can do whatever feels great for your body in this pose too. Stretch back to child's pose, move around in circles, or move your torso like a jump rope — just play with what feels amazing and necessary in your body.

Downward Dog

From tabletop, place your feet farther back and come into downward dog pose in which your legs and arms are straightish and your butt is in the air. Peddle your legs, gently stretching your hamstrings and sides. Concentrate on the inhale and the exhale. Be gentle. Any pain is a sign to stop.

The kind of stress that nurses endure is bewildering to me. We are constantly bombarded with strangers and their emotions: anger, rage, happiness, sadness, confusion, or shame. Yoga is a simple practice that can help you to release, get centered, and increase your capacity to be kind to strangers. All these practices are steps toward preventing you from becoming a fried and crispy nurse.

Day 11

Advocating for Your Patients

I had been collaborating with the doctor to get our patient's terminal agitation under control; it took us two hours. The family had finally settled into their chairs, and the patient began to exhibit Cheyne-Stokes respirations signaling the end was near. The family requested to speak to the doctor. The physician went into the room and came back 10 minutes later. He was a little pale and said, "The patient died while I was in there. I have never been in the room with someone when they died."

I thought, "You have *never* been with a patient when they died?" I was struck by what an excellent hospice doctor he was despite this. In that same moment, I suddenly realized the powerful role of the bedside nurse. I had been with hundreds of patients and families at the patient's bedside while they were dying. I have a critical vantage point. We are bedside nurses, but we are also witnesses, advocates, and activists for our patients.

Self-Care Practice

Today's practice will be a reflection practice to consider how we can advocate for nurses because when we advocate for nurses, we are advocating for our patients.

For the next 20 minutes, you are going to do a little dreaming in your journal. This is to get you excited about possibilities, not to weigh you down with the realities. Consider and reflect on the following.

Research on compassion reveals that compassionate care improves patient outcomes. When nurses feel physically safe, emotionally supported, and are not overwhelmed by inadequate staffing ratios, they can deliver compassionate care to their patients. When medicine is delivered with compassion, it builds trust between the patient and clinician. When the patient trusts the nurse, they share more information and nuances about their illness and adhere to the medical advice and treatment. When the appropriate treatment is chosen and the patient adheres to medical advice, their outcomes improve (Vachon, 2020). When there is ample time to assess your patient *and* chart, nurses can leave on time and skip home knowing they have time for something else today — anything else. Everyone wins. The patient wins, the clinician wins, and the community wins.

Reflect on how the nurses in your unit could improve *the way* they give care. What could spark more compassion? Do they need more time to assess? To chart? To admit? To discharge? Is there something you can ask for? Is it better staffing ratios, more CNAs, a unit secretary, or adequate PPE? Better training? More training? Any training at all? You get the idea.

Dream big — we have to start somewhere.

Dream a little more: What processes are in place that are working? What is not working? Do you have detailed checklists for discharges or admits? How can the handoffs be improved? How are the relationships with the CNAs? How are the relationships between the evening shift, the night shift, and the day shift?[11]

Are there opportunities for nurses to get involved? Is there a shared governance committee? Is there a union? Have you been to a nurse meeting lately?

Listen, I am not a manager or administrator — I just do not know who is going to appropriately advocate for nurses except for nurses. The nurse plays a critical and powerful role in patient care and outcomes. Yes, you are advocating for yourself, but in the end, you are advocating for your patients.

---

11   This is often an area that requires a little more grace from all shifts. Every shift has their cons: The day shift must navigate the discharges, breakfast and lunch, teams of professionals, specialists, families, extended families, etc. The evening shift gets the admissions, the sundowners, the full-moon antics, dinner, and the harried family members who arrive after work. The night shift must call the exhausted doctors in the middle of the night, let the patient sleep while inserting Foleys and IVs, dress wounds, and deal with the unit ghosts — all in the dark. When I would hand off to my evening shift colleague Julie and say, "I am sorry, but I didn't get to complete the XYZ," she would say. "No worries, that's the beauty of 24/7 care. I got you, BC." So graceful.

Day 12

Just One Intentional Minute

I waited tables during college in a Mexican-inspired, ruffly dress. I raced around the restaurant carrying trays so wide they could hardly squeeze through the double swinging kitchen doors and so heavy that after three months my right arm was noticeably larger than my left. I like to think I was smooth with customers, laughing, engaging them, and listening to their stories while the back of my brain was spinning: "guacamole to Table 6, taquitos to Table 7, and four margaritas, one with no salt, to Table 8."

I found nursing weirdly similar without the ruffles or margaritas. I ran from room to room in my sensible shoes with my stethoscope draped around my neck, carrying flushes, a pen light, IV bags, and catheter kits. I stopped to engage with the patients and the families, asking questions about their symptoms while charting or lightly bantering with one foot out the door while the back of my brain was spinning with orders:

"morphine in Room 5, IV vancomycin in Room 6, stop the drip in Room 7, dressing change in Room 8."

Most patients and families can feel when you are busy and distracted on those hectic days (which is, um, every day).

I began a practice of sitting next to my patient's bedside, asking open ended questions, and timing it. I found that even one minute of presence and openness was a game changer — the energy shifts for everyone.[12] The patient and family relax and open up more. I could gather more information by taking in the nuances of the family dynamics or the patient's overall being. I felt that some days sitting with them palliated them more than trying to answer their unanswerable questions or medicating them with Ativan.

Demonstrating therapeutic presence to a patient by really listening to them, even for just a minute, has been found to facilitate the healing process in patients and gives them emotional energy to deal with their illness (Vachon, 2020).

Self-Care Practice

Nurses are taskmasters; with too many patients and endless charting, you always have something you should be doing. Today, you are going to practice not doing anything. Do not worry, research has shown this will not kill you.[13]

Find a comfortable seat — ideally in a space where you like to spend a lot of time. If you want, you can play some nice

---

[12] I learned this presence by watching my nurse mentors at Hopewell House, a beautiful hospice home in Portland, Oregon.

[13] I know this to be true after years of watching my family lie around on weekends.

background music. Sit in a comfortable chair, on the couch, or the floor. Set your timer for 10 minutes, and play with what it feels like to not do anything.

Feel your body in the chair, take some breaths, and notice if there is any tension in your body. Take in the sights and the sounds of the room without getting up and putting the debris away. *There is that big pile of bills. Is that the refrigerator humming? There is my cat.* Keep breathing. Try to relax into the chair. Look at the pattern in the carpet, the color of the walls, or the plants.

Note what comes up for you as you practice stillness and presence.

When you are still, open, and breathing during your nursing shift, even for a minute, patients and their families are less stressed. They know they have time to ask questions, and you begin the process of developing rapport and trust. Your intentional presence allows more space to tune into the physical subtleties and overall energy of the room. Let the physical, emotional, and spiritual healing begin.

Day 13

Pie

On those days that we felt the burden of staff cuts, new Medicare regulations, and charting laws, my co-worker Suzy and I would dream about opening a pie shop. We imagined rising bright and early thinking about fruit and flaky crusts. We imagined flour and brown sugar covering our cute aprons while laughing all day. We could just focus on pies and making our customers happy. No charting, no insurance, no broken families, no sputum on your scrubs, no waiting for test results, no death, and no grief. Just pie.

Some days you may dream about working in a pie shop or a desk job where you can internet shop all day, but there are not many professions where you can assist a woman giving birth, help someone walk again, bring a patient's pain level from a 10 to a zero, or support a patient through cancer treatment and recovery. These patients need you. Desperately. People do not desperately need pie.

Well, maybe some days they do.

Self-Care Practice

It is normal that healthcare providers become periodically emotionally exhausted and want to leave their professions. Typically, after a period of rest and renewal, though, the privilege of doing this work re-emerges and the desire to help others returns (Vachon, 2020).

You have met the crunchy nurse that is a little grumpy and the one that is ambivalent, not giving a whoopty-f**king-doo.[14] It takes some practice to intentionally recharge your spirit. Reflect for the next 20 minutes on what rest and renewal could look like for you. You can review the self-care practices that you have tried while working through this book. Perhaps you need to do absolutely nothing some days. Or maybe baking a pie can recharge your soul. Do you need a day off? A weekend away? A sabbatical? Just dream.

I worked in short-stay surgery, and I loved it for six years. Suddenly, though, I did not love it. I felt like I needed a break and a period to relax, spend time with my three kids, and discern what was next. My co-workers would say, "Beth, don't do it. This is the best nursing job you will ever find. No weekends, no holidays, home by 3 p.m." They had a point, but I felt like my heart was not in it anymore. I quit with a nine-month time frame in my head, a gestation period. I spent time with my

---

14 Vachon describes this emotional detachment as an "easy defense against emotional exhaustion," but it negatively impacts the clinician's personal life, relationships, mental health, and patient outcomes (Vachon, 2020, pp. 312–317). Also, "whoopty-f**king-doo" is not his term, just for the record.

husband and family, I walked slowly to the library with my kids, and we ate ice cream in the front yard every sunny day.

When I went back to work, I decided to work on call at a gorgeous hospice home, which became my life's work for the next 15 years. Spirit recharged.[15]

---

15 I know most nurses cannot just quit their jobs, but we have options: on call, per diem, nights or day shift, short-stay surgery, hospice, cardiac care, travel nursing, administration, teaching, or phone triage. My restless spirit loves the variety.

Day 14

Super-Friggin Hero

In the spring of 2020, health care workers were finally given the title they deserve: *hero*. I unscientifically polled my colleagues, and their feelings about this word were mixed. Some felt that this word was BS rhetoric dissuading the staff from quitting, others felt undeserving of the term because they were not on the front lines enough, and some said, "Hell yes, I am a super-friggin hero."

Although I had just quit my job at the time, I was ecstatic about the word *hero* being attributed to nurses during the pandemic — nursing is an intense job and always has been. Nursing requires brains, brute strength, and benevolence. You speed walk from room to room, and sprinting is not uncommon. You lift and hoist heavy objects and fragile humans who are often difficult to move with lines, drains, and pins holding their body parts together. You offer deep compassion while your patient is explosively vomiting into the emesis basin you are holding. You bear witness to suffering mothers and fathers who cannot possibly bear the news that their child has cancer. You can insert IVs, Foleys, and rectal tubes while discussing the weather. And somehow you look into the patient's soul *while* you are charting. You perform these tasks gracefully, tenderly, and yes, heroically, in the midst of chaos and fear. You did all of this *before* the pandemic.

You did not graduate from nursing school with these emotional skills of composure and tenderness while the s**t is hitting the fan — or the floor. The science of compassion shows that groundedness, rootedness, composure, and grace while under pressure come from years of practice and training (Vachon, 2020).

Self-Care Practice

To boost your ability to be composed, grounded, and compassionate while caring for sick patients, the science of compassion reveals that you can develop practices to train your mind. Today's self-care practice offers a beginner's guide to meditation. Meditation is the practice of trying to still your mind.

Find a comfortable position in a quiet room. Set a timer for 10 minutes. Next, focus on your breath. You can pay attention to the inhale and the exhale or the rise and fall of your chest. Your job is to focus on your breath for the next 10 minutes.

Your thoughts will come and go — notice them without judgment and without following the thought. They will continue to come and go — they may get loud, and they may yell to "*just empty the dishwasher!*" Simply notice and bring your attention back to the breath. No one is a perfect meditator, so there is no striving for perfection. The goal is to notice when you are following your thoughts and then bring your attention back to the breath with compassion — each time, every time, hundreds of times.

Over time, you will notice an inner stillness developing that will help you to feel renewed in the long term, but today, you simply have to devote 10 minutes to this one practice of paying attention to your breath.[16]

---

16 I will admit I am not a great meditator when I am all alone in a room. I have found myself looking in the fridge for a snack in the middle of my 10-minute meditation. I can sustain a seated posture longer if I listen to a guided meditation, especially one by Tara Brach.

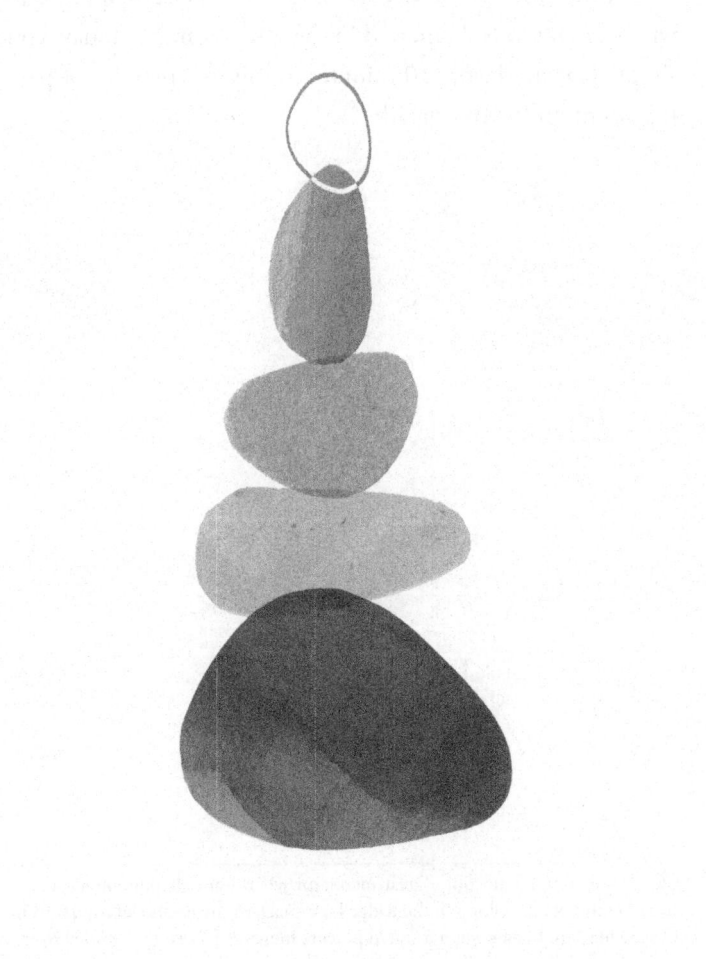

Day 15

No No No No No

Rumination is when we let a problem, a thought, or an event play repeatedly in our mind. As a nurse, this is quite easy for me to do. My dear brother-in-law Jeff died from ALS, and I was with him the day he died. I repositioned him with my husband, gave him Ativan, and helped my sister wash his face. He was unresponsive, and the hospice nurse said he had somewhere between hours and days to live.

I am not sure if I avoided it, did not believe it, or if he really did not appear imminent, but our family drove away from the house. We received a call four hours later that he died. I was shocked and frustrated that we did not stay. I could not get this out of my head. What signs did I miss? Why did I not see it coming? I should have known better. I should have stayed. I continually played the scene in my head wondering how I, an experienced hospice nurse, missed this.

The challenge of a ruminating mind is often underestimated

and can be quite distressing. We tend to ruminate on the negative — our mistakes, our fears, and our anxieties.

Self-Care Practice

The following exercise is a practical tool developed by MJ Murray Vachon that can help you to pause and shift your rumination. Murray Vachon describes ruminating thoughts as "intrusive and at times haunting, which means even when we are focusing on something else, they tend to be spinning in the back of our mind, likely causing some physiological distress."

Find a quiet space. Bring a pen, a notebook, and some snacks.

1. Is there a work scenario or job frustration that you keep replaying in your head? Take some time to write this down in detail.

2. Is your story accurate? Is it the entire story? Sometimes we make up a story about the event, and often, we fill in the gaps if we do not know the entire story. Write about this.

3. Focus on what you are *feeling* at this moment and *where* in your body these emotional sensations are located. Sometimes this is obvious; other times we need a bit of patience to locate where our feelings have landed.

4. Now sit with these uncomfortable feelings, take a few breaths, and imagine breathing them out of your body. Even though it is counterintuitive to hold pain, it can be helpful to do so. You can imagine breathing your feelings into a container or into the ocean.

5. Reconsider this work scenario or job frustration. Notice if your mind is more open to new thoughts and information about this situation. Pay attention to those that are more positive. Write these thoughts down.

6. Notice how, if given a bit of time and attention, your brain can naturally shift to more positive information that makes the story you are telling yourself not so worrisome, negative, or catastrophic. Allow yourself to sit with this shift and breathe through it for as long as necessary.

7. Pay attention if an action plan begins to surface in your mind. An action plan is an antidote to rumination. It helps us move from being stuck in fear to doing something that can help resolve the situation or accept it without being self-critical or afraid. There are no limits to an appropriate action plan. Sometimes it is sleep, an apology, or a commitment to better communication. Often a common action plan is being kinder and gentler with yourself. Maybe it is as simple as reminding yourself that we are human and will make mistakes. Most ruminations have a bit of truth in them, but the negative bias of our fears can paralyze us and distort our perceptions.

8. Take your action plan and run a movie of yourself carrying out the plan in your mind — the more detailed the better. Rehearse it. Do this three times. (Yes, you are now ruminating on your action plan.)

9. You may need to run through your action plan throughout the day or week until you can carry it out. This

process helps strengthen your ability to work through ruminations. Trust that you have done what you can for now and get on with your day. Do the dishes, listen to music, or go to work. Just do not feed the rumination by talking about it with others or letting your mind spin.

Day 16

A Soft, Fluffy, Edgy Nurse

Most nurses have a bit of an edge, even the soft, fluffy ones. This edge allows you to eat your lunch after you complete the most unimaginable procedure or laugh with your co-worker right before you plunge your hands into some rashy, edematous crevice. This edge is necessary for your professional survival.

This edge is also necessary for your patient's survival. You know what it takes to heal the patient and get them home. Often this involves performing uncomfortable clinical procedures and pushing the patient to get out of bed, walk, take their medication, do their knee exercises, drink more fluids, eat, or poop. You educate, you motivate, and you inspire. This edge is a helpful tool that allows you to also see through the BS, to not be manipulated, and to advocate for your patients. Compassion science reveals that compassion is not a sentimentalized soft attitude; rather, compassion is the ability to do what is needed for the ultimate benefit of the patient (Vachon, 2020). I love nurses. Nurses are a perfect blend of warrior and angel.

Self-Care Practice

Today's practice will focus on the subtleties of the mind-body connection and our masculine-feminine polarities. This is a practice I learned and adapted from Tami Kent, physical therapist, energy healer, and women's holistic pelvic-care practitioner (Kent, 2014).

Find a quiet space. Take a comfortable seat or lie down. Sense where your body connects with the ground. Take some deep breaths and focus your attention on your pelvic area, approximately where your ovaries are or would be located.

Now focus your attention on the right side of your pelvic area. The right side is our masculine side — our doer, organizer, planner, goal-oriented, taskmaster side. My guess is most nurses live most of their days in the right side of their energetic body — doing, running, planning, triaging, organizing, and calculating. Take some breaths and sense into this space. Do you feel any sensations arising from this side of your body? Numbness, tingling, space, or density? Just notice.

Now visualize taking some breaths to fluff up the energy in this side of your pelvis, and ask your body: What do I need? Listen for the response. It may be a simple word like *sleep*, *rest*, *water*, *food*, or *change*, or it may be an image that leads you to a specific action or desire.

Give thanks to your masculine side for all that it does.

Now focus on the left side of your pelvis. Take some breaths and sense into this space. This is your feminine side — your intuitive, sensitive, creative, connected, playful side. What do you notice? Nothing? Numbness, density, coolness, a yearning, quiet, space, or heat? Take some breaths and imagine creating energetic space here. Ask the question: What do I need? It may be one simple word or a quick image of paints, a bookstore, quiet, meditation, or a nap. Give thanks to your intuitive wisdom.

Now take some breaths and imagine that center line that runs down your body softening, blending, and connecting these two sides of you. Pay attention to anything that comes to mind: images, colors, or sensations. Be open and aware as you breathe.

When you learn to inhabit your body in a different way, it can shift things for you mentally, physically, and energetically. This exercise is a way to restore balance while listening to and trusting your body. Nurses have professional intuitive instincts. This practice involves paying attention to subtleties and nuances in your body. You are simply honing your craft while cultivating mindful awareness of the needs of your own warrior and your angel.

Write or draw about this experience.

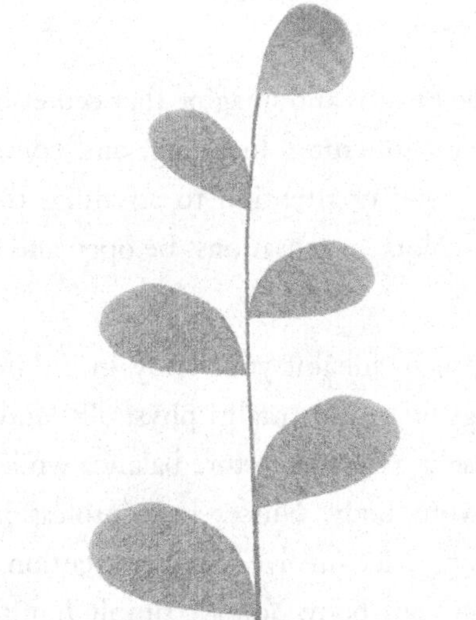

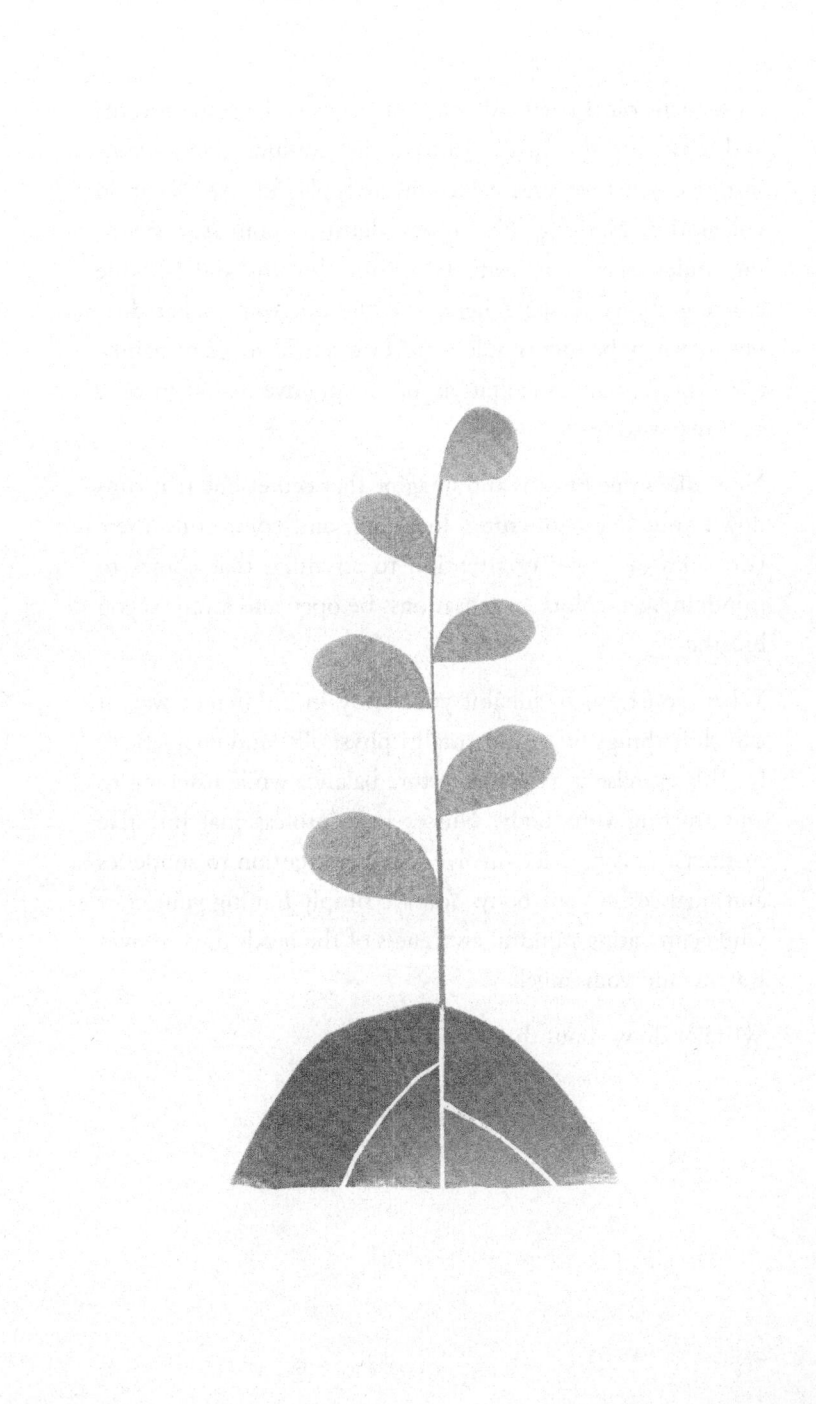

Day 17

Marshmallows and Peanut Butter

Most shifts in health care are ridiculously busy. One hospice shift stands out for me. Out of my five patients, one needed aggressive med titration for pain, one needed to be weaned from 30 liters of O2, and another had a sudden terminal event. Two of my patients died on that shift. I also needed to support many emotionally fragile family members, and I never ate my lunch.[17]

I picked up my kids from their elementary school and hauled them into the grocery store to find some avocados and chicken. Once I arrived at home, I threw the kids some marshmallows and peanut butter and loudly started dinner while clutching my glass of wine.

---

[17] Not eating lunch is a terrible idea but a common experience. This is another cultural shift needed in nursing.

Self-Care Practice

Transitioning from work to home is particularly startling. Your home life requires completely different skill sets and energy than your work life. Like high performance athletes, clinicians need rituals and regular practices that give their bodies and minds time to recover from hard work and allow effortless rest (Loehr & Schwartz, 2003; Vachon, 2020).

It is important for health care professionals to create grounding rituals and routines in their daily life, so they can become habitually re-energized.

Write down some ideas for a five-to-30-minute ritual to help you shift gears after work. You want it to feel effortless but intentional. Commit to one of these after your next shift.

Here are some examples of a gear-shifting practice:

- Rain or shine, take a 15-minute walk when you arrive home.
- Listen to a five-minute mindfulness meditation while driving home from work.
- Take off your scrubs with care, bless them, and throw them, as hard as you can, into the washing machine.
- Take a quick shower and visualize all the frantic hospital energy from your shift (your patients, families, and co-workers) being washed away into the drain.
- Bike home from work (this also requires that you bike to work, which could also be a good pre-shift ritual).

- Lie down on the floor for 15 minutes and let those 15 minutes matter. Breathe, feel the work tension, honor it, then release it.

Experiment with different ones until you find the one that eases your transition from work to home.

Day 18

How Care Is Delivered

The science of compassion research shows that when medicine is delivered in a compassionate way it enhances the treatment and improves patient outcomes. If medicine is delivered in an uncaring, purely technical way, it can have negative outcomes (Vachon, 2020).

Compassion *should be* the driver in medical care.[18]

I have the honor of working with extraordinary nurses. One nurse named Libby comes to mind. I walked past a patient's room and saw Libby helping a frail adult patient out of bed. A few minutes later I walked past again, and the patient was holding tightly to Libby's waist — it looked like they were slow dancing. They both looked at me and smiled. I kid you not, a minute later this patient had wrapped her arms around Libby and was hugging her like a tender grandma. Libby hugged her back.

---

18 Not profit. Not insurance payments. Not Medicare regulations.

I know and feel the pain of being a nurse. It is a stressful job with too much to do all the time. It is hard some days to find any morsel of compassion. Here is the good news: You can train yourself to be compassionate. And I say that because I did not really become compassionate until I worked at it while being mentored by the awesome nurses around me.[19]

Self-Care Practice

It is important to develop practices that help to maintain your compassion, composure, and unwavering unflappability. Various forms of meditation can help train one's mind for this work. Today, practice the following loving kindness meditation to enhance your compassionate mindset. This adaptation of a loving kindness meditation can be done from a Buddhist or secular perspective (Salzberg, 2002; Halifax et al., 2007). Neuroscience research shows it is beneficial for both patients and clinicians (Vachon, 2020; Weng et al., 2017).

Find a quiet place and take a comfortable seat. Take some deep breaths to ground yourself in the moment, your space, and your body.

Choose someone in your life whom you find *easy to love*. It might be a spouse, a child, or a safe bet like your cat or dog. Imagine their face in front of you and how you feel when you are with them. Fixate on this feeling in your heart for a few minutes. Do not worry if your mind drifts off. Gently bring your attention back to your breath and then to your heart center again.

---

19 This began when I worked at a hospice home called Hopewell House in Portland, Oregon, in 2006.

Now, still imagining this person's or pet's face in front of you, speak or silently offer the following phrases to your easy-to-love chosen one, pausing between each line:

May you be happy.

May you be safe.

May you be free from suffering.

Take some deep breaths, and feel the warm glow in your body these phrases evoke. Just be with this feeling. Compassion is a muscle, and it needs to be strengthened. This is a way to lengthen and contract this muscle.

Now think of a neutral person — maybe the FedEx delivery person or the grocery store greeter. Picture them in front of you, and wish them well:

May you be happy.

May you be safe.

May you be free from suffering.

Take a few minutes and think about that delivery person. Of course, they should be happy and safe. Why not wish them that? This practice helps us feel compassionately for everyone, even those you do not have a significant relationship with.

Then think about yourself. Place your hand on your heart and whisper the following:

May I be happy.

May I be safe.

May I be free from suffering.

Yes. This is a difficult practice for many, but if the Fed Ex person can be happy, then of course you should be free from suffering too!

You may need to work up to the next part of the meditation. Seriously, it is OK if you are not there yet. This is a practice, not a perfection. For the next step in this loving kindness meditation, consider someone that you find difficult to be in relationship with. Is there a co-worker that is particularly tough to work with or a family member that continues to frustrate you? Take some breaths, imagine their face, and slowly offer these same wishes:

May you be happy.

May you be safe.

May you be free from suffering.

This loving kindness meditation is a sweet reminder that everyone deserves to be happy, safe, and free from suffering while decreasing your heart rate and your blood pressure. Loving kindness also can shift your mental outlook and help to develop and maintain your compassionate mindset so you can deliver your unwavering kindness and medical care to *all* your patients, even the tricky ones.

Day 19

Dirty Children

Some days, you will not feel like a superhero. You get home from work and bypass the loads of laundry, the takeout containers in the fridge, the unpaid bills, and crash on the couch to watch "Game of Thrones" with your children. When you see the advertisements praising nurses as heroes, you may want to scream: "I am not a hero! I am a human. I cried at work today, my fridge is a mess, my children have not showered, and I have a urinary tract infection. Heroes do not get UTIs." Sometimes, the cape feels like a heavy burden.

I am here to tell you that people do not think you are perfect; they think you are relatable. The celebration of you honors your commitment to the health and wellness of our community. Every one of your shifts positively impacts another person's life. Now that you are home, you do not have to take care of everyone perfectly. You know firsthand that our bodies are capable of surviving cancer and kidney stones. Your kids will endure another showerless day.

Self-Care Practice

Humility, altruism, and generosity are beautiful characteristics that plague most nurses I know. I want you to get comfortable for the next 20 minutes as you reflect on your compassion satisfaction, the pleasure and satisfaction you feel when you help someone else. This simple but profound task will help you to deal with stress and protect you from burnout (Vachon, 2020).

Take 20 minutes to journal.

Lean into those good, juicy stories from your recent shifts, big and small. What are some moments where you positively impacted a patient — alleviating respiratory distress, the successful and rapid titration of pain meds, or the satisfaction you felt when you inserted the urinary catheter and drained a liter.

Consider how lucky you are to be with a patient during the most intimate and fragile moments of their lives — as they grapple with their kidney failure, during their first round of chemo, or while they reunite with their son. What does it feel like to support these intimate moments with your care? These stories might fill your heart with sparkly rainbows, puffy clouds, and unicorns. When you focus on the positive stories and the privilege of your profession, this will help prevent you from burning out.

Day 20

Sparkles in the Carpet

One day, after being so kind and gentle to all my dying patients, their family members, and my co-workers, I came home, and my husband was lying face down on the living room floor sleeping while our three kids covered the carpet with rainbow sprinkles. Their faces and hands had sticky rainbow remnants. "Mama, it's so pretty!" Grace said enthusiastically as they all licked their hands. All my compassion and kindness flew out the door. My blood boiled at my husband's perceived laziness as I considered the next hour of vacuuming and bathing of children.

I fake smiled, walked upstairs, and quietly threw a tube of disgusting blue toothpaste against our white bedroom wall. It was a little disturbing to me that I could be so kind to my patients but sometimes give my husband so little room to be human. I hopped into the shower, took some breaths, gathered myself together, and walked past the blue sludge on the wall to join my family downstairs.

Working in health care requires intense mental and emotional work. Most people present their best selves at work and have little left when they land at home. Clinicians must take the time to tend to their close relationships (Vachon, 2020).

Close relationships are like owning a car. You cannot just hop into it and expect it to run forever. You have to clean it, fill it with gas often, get the lube/oil/filter changed every 5,000 miles or so, replace the brake pads when they wear down, and rotate the tires. A relationship requires ongoing maintenance.

Self-Care Practice

For today's practice, you will consider your critical relationships in your life and how you can tend to one of them. This exercise is not intended to beat yourself up about the should haves and would haves. You are going to have a growth mindset with this one and meet yourself with compassion and love.

Write down the names of your important people.

Choose one relationship. Now brainstorm some ways you can tend to this person today, and then follow it up with an action. It can be as simple as a phone call, making them a cup of tea, or lying next to them face down on the carpet while the kids shower you with sprinkles. One intentional moment will not fix a neglected relationship, but awareness combined with action is a step toward maintaining or healing your relationships.

Day 21

Hoist, Hustle, Hurdle

Being in health care is physically challenging. One shift may be equivalent to an Olympic triathlon without the medal, orange slices, or cheering crowds. There is so much squatting, lifting, running, walking, hustling, sprinting, hurdling, hoisting, bending, pulling, and pushing involved in nursing. Even with the best training and ergonomic intentions, nurses can get themselves into some awkward positions.

I was helping a gentleman get dressed and put on his slippers. He had a walker in front of him, his nonskid socks were on, the aide was to his side, and I was in front, squatting next to his feet about to assist him with his shoes. We had every fall precaution in place and two smart women right next to him. Everything happened so fast and slowly at the same time. Our patient suddenly fell backward. I lurched forward instinctively to grab him and felt my back go *zingggggg*. Our patient landed with a thud. We assessed him, and thankfully, he had no injuries other than a bruised ego. The rest of the shift, my back felt like it was on fire as I contemplated possible nurse desk jobs. Luckily, I awoke the next day feeling fine. Phew.

I do not think people have a clue about the amount of brawn that is necessary to be a successful nurse. And by successful, I mean a nurse who is not injured.

Every time I hoist a patient up in bed with an aide or volunteer, I pray they have the same strength I do. When a patient is a "one-person assist" and I am the one assisting them to the commode or toilet, I pray this is not the day their legs give out.

Difficult work over the long haul requires that clinicians must take time to care for themselves physically, mentally, and spiritually. The long-term temptation in dealing with suffering in others is to not care for yourself (Vachon, 2020).

Self- Care Practice

For today's practice, you will do a body scan.

Find a quiet comfortable space. I always do these lying down, but you can do this practice sitting in a chair as well.

As you do the body scan, inhale and notice any types of sensation you experience — tingling, awareness, tension, warmth, or heaviness. When you exhale, imagine that part of your body and the surrounding muscles releasing.

You may want to spend extra breaths in certain areas of your body that feel particularly tense.

Start at the top of your head and work your way down to your toes.

Take some deep, full-body breaths.

As you inhale, bring attention to your head. As you exhale, let your head get heavy and feel supported.

On the next inhale, move to your eyes. Take a long deep exhale and allow the muscles around your eyes to soften.

Now focus on the space between your ears. On the inhale, notice if there is any tension. On the exhale, allow this space to expand a bit.

Move your awareness to your jaw — this area will require a few breaths. Gently and tenderly move your jaw and with each exhale, allow it to unhinge a bit.

Continue to move down each part of your body. Intentionally inhale and exhale slowly while noticing the tension and offering any release.

Move to:

> Your throat
>
> The back of your neck
>
> Your shoulders
>
> The front of your heart space
>
> Your upper back
>
> Your belly
>
> Your lower back
>
> Your hips and the space between your hips
>
> Your thighs

Your knees

Your shins and calves

Your ankles

And finally, to your feet.

Continue to breathe with your whole-body awareness while paying attention to any sensations that arise.

Nurses pay an inordinate amount of attention to their patient's body parts. It is important to offer yourself that same attention.

Day 22

Healing Touch

Nurses are in constant physical contact with patients, and it is easy to forget how profound this is. My friend was admitted to the hospital during a shelter-in-place order for the pandemic. As her nurses and doctors performed routine tasks — listening to her heart, helping her change into a gown, pulling her up in bed — she was struck by how much she missed being touched. She believed, in fact, that this "routine" touch was one of the most important aspects to her healing.

There are not many professions that allow for this type of intimacy with people — it is an honor and a privilege. Jean Watson's theory of caring states that when nurses "reverentially assist with basic needs as sacred acts, they are touching the mind/body/spirit of another, (thereby sustaining) their human dignity" (Watson, 2021). This intentionality fosters the patient's physical, emotional, and spiritual healing.

Self-Care Practice

Reflect on the myriad of ways you touch your patients: dressing a wound, repositioning a patient, changing a patient's briefs, assisting them out of bed, listening to their heart and lungs, palpating their abdomen, and feeling for edema in the lower extremities. Because of this professional intimacy, you have this amazing opportunity to show care for your patients.

I have been on the receiving end of hospital staff before, and let me tell you, there is a difference between intentional touch and performing a rote procedure. I have felt cared for, and I have also had the experience of feeling violated. When I have not felt cared for, I shut down and did not trust the clinician.

Consider some commitments you can make around how you care for your patients. These should not add any time to your shift or tasks but rather increase your intentionality in the moment. Maybe commit to remove dressings slowly or to tenderly lift your patient's head when you flip the pillow. Leave your hand on your patient's shoulder when you listen to their heart or rub their back when they lean forward in bed as you listen to their lungs.

Nursing can be incredibly intimate, and every time we touch our patients, they should be treated with reverence, respect, and kindness. These simple moments can foster their healing while increasing your job satisfaction.[20]

---

20 Jean Watson asserts that the patient-nurse relationship is mutually beneficial. When nurses touch their patients with respect and dignity, nurses are being touched and healed in the same moment (Watson, 2021).

Day 23

Simple Gestures Lead to the Sacred

After the death of one of my patients, the family and I cleaned his body, applied lavender lotion, and dressed him from head to toe with a button-down shirt, belt, hat, and glasses — the whole deal. He looked as if he was ready to go to work when we finished. Family photos were placed on his bedside table next to a battery-operated candle. We then called in the chaplain, who said a prayer over his body. We placed flowers on his chest and a beautiful quilt over his body, keeping his face exposed. End-of-life rituals are deeply healing.

Self-Care Practice

Clinicians need rituals or regular practices that give their bodies and minds time to recover from hard work (Loehr & Schwartz, 2003; Vachon, 2020). Perhaps you have been practicing a transition-from-work-to-home ritual since Day 17.

Today, we are going to add to that.

Create a sacred area in your home that helps you ground and connect with your inner life. This is your go-to place when you need some inspiration and a quiet space to recover from this difficult work. It could be on your bedside table, a corner of the living room, or the guest bedroom. If you already have one, add to it. Do you have a favorite flower, a book of poetry, or meaningful photos? Add any elements of nature that make you smile, including stones, branches, or leaves. How about sage or a fragrant candle? Maybe add art supplies, a journal, or a divine statue. When you are done, bless this space as a holy one, whatever that means to you. Return to this space whenever you need to fluff up your weary soul.

Day 24

Divine Flow

My nursing profession has always informed my spiritual journey. Early on, I declared the hospice home my church — it was in this special building that I experienced a sacred connection with my patients and their families and felt a powerful holy presence. I discovered that I could get in *the flow* on my shifts — I would often feel moved and compelled by a divine force.[21]

One night shift when I arrived at work, the nurse said to me at report, "Our patient in Room 7 is transitioning, but not actively dying. Don't call her father in because he just left at 9 p.m. He's old and frail and flew in today from Chicago." So, we checked on this patient, who was 40 — my age at the

---

[21] I kept this to myself until I read Vachon's book. He freely discusses the divine flow and clinicians' spiritual experiences while at work. He writes, "There are times when everything they know comes together in a way that flows easily and powerfully, and they are even astonished with the intuition and wisdom that comes out of their own mouths" (Vachon, 2020, p. 488). It is a thing.

time. She looked peaceful. Her respirations were faint but regular. Her pulses were stable but thready. After 30 minutes, I went back into the room and sat near her bed. Although it was midnight and she showed no clinical signs of actively dying, I felt compelled to call her father back in. He arrived at 1 a.m., physically supported by younger relatives. Initially, part of me regretted waking him because he was so frail.

He sat next to his daughter's bedside and rested his hand on hers. I would come in throughout the night and sit on the other side of her bed. He stayed in that chair all night, intermittently dozing and rousing when I entered the room. He shared sweet stories about his daughter and tenderly discussed her life as an adult. It was a holy night for him. His daughter did not change drastically throughout the night but slipped away, dying peacefully at 7 a.m. with her father holding her hand.

As I processed her beautiful death, it became clear to me that even if the patient had died two days later, her father would never regret that time at her bedside. He was given that special and quiet time to be with her, to grieve, to share stories, to mourn, and to hold vigil. I am glad I listened to my instincts and called him up. This death has informed many of my future choices about when to call in family members. I am now much more open to nuances, intuition, and something bigger than vital signs.

Self-Care Practice

Research on the science of compassion reveals that reflecting on your philosophy of life or your sense of spirituality can help you recover from this difficult work. Vachon writes, "There must be a constant connection with one's purpose and mission so that one can stay motivated … and be able to bounce back from setbacks and mistakes and tragic situations" (Vachon, 2020, p. 493). Reflecting on my spirituality calms that persistent question that often arises in the hospital: "What is this all for?"

Today, you will spend the next 20 minutes sitting with or reflecting on your spirituality or philosophy of life.[22] Consider these questions:

How do you reconcile the events you see on your shifts with your greater understanding of life? Do you ever have the sense that there is some intangible force at work or something greater than yourself? Do you receive any gifts from your patient stories or work experiences?

Ponder the mystery of being human — our fragility and our strength. You spend so much time in your head. Think about the experiences that tap into your heart. When do you notice your intuition is accurate while at work or otherwise? Do you experience profound moments that take your breath away?

Your growth as a clinician is not static — it is an ongoing series of awakenings (Vachon, 2020).

Thank goodness.

---

[22] Vachon has an elegant list of questions that helps clinicians articulate their SOC/POC (spirituality of caring/philosophy of caring) to find deeper satisfaction in their work. See Vachon, 2020, pp. 485–486.

Day 25

Am I Dying?

I took care of a patient who was on a ventilator in the hospital, weaned from the vent, and came to the hospice home I was working at to die. She arrived unresponsive with multiple tear-stained family members. We gently prepped the family for her death and emotionally supported them.

Two days later, the patient's eyelids fluttered open. I was readjusting her position as the granddaughter sat knitting in the corner of the room. The patient looked around and weakly asked if she was in the hospital. I told her she was indeed very sick. Then she asked if she was dying. I pulled up a chair and said, "Yes, the doctors think you are dying. You were on a ventilator for a week. They weaned you off it, and you came to the hospice house to die. We are going to keep you comfortable, and your granddaughter is here."

This patient suddenly looked angry and glared at her granddaughter: "I am at the hospice house again?" I had no idea she had been here before. I suddenly had the feeling this woman was not going to follow doctor's orders.

Veracity is being completely truthful with patients — nurses must not withhold the whole truth from clients, even if it may lead to patient distress. I love that ethical principles are woven into our nursing profession, providing structure and rigor to the field. Although uncomfortable, I pulled up a chair and told this woman we all indeed thought she was dying.

The patient was distressed, and yet, she did not die. I think that information helped her to gather all the strength and will she could muster to get the heck out of the hospice house. She left our hospice a week later and went on to live her life.

Self-Care Practice

The ethical foundations of nursing have become much more meaningful to me after being a nurse for a while. I now lean on them daily to explain the benefits and burdens of IV fluids, the proper use of opioids, or what it looks like to wean a patient off oxygen. We have to take a neutral stance as we offer our patients and families information to make decisions about their health. Then we must honor and advocate for whatever decision they make.

- Justice is fairness. Nurses must be fair when they distribute care, for example, among the patients in the group of patients that they are taking care of. Care must be fairly, justly, and equitably distributed among a group of patients.
- Beneficence is doing good and the right thing for the patient.

- Nonmaleficence is doing no harm, as stated in the historical Hippocratic Oath. Harm can be intentional or unintentional.

- Accountability is accepting responsibility for one's own actions. Nurses are accountable for their nursing care and other actions. They must accept all the professional and personal consequences that can occur as the result of their actions.

- Veracity is being completely truthful with patients; nurses must not withhold the whole truth from clients even when it may lead to patient distress.

- Fidelity is keeping one's promises. The nurse must be faithful and true to their professional promises and responsibilities by providing high-quality, safe care in a competent manner.

- Autonomy and patient self-determination are upheld when the nurse accepts the client as a unique person who has the innate right to have their own opinions, perspectives, values, and beliefs. Nurses encourage patients to make their own decisions without any judgments or coercion from the nurse. The patient has the right to reject or accept all treatments.

Nursing is a noble profession. You are equal parts educator and advocate. You are a steward of resources and equitable access to health care. You value truth, faithfulness, and justice. Let us keep it that way.

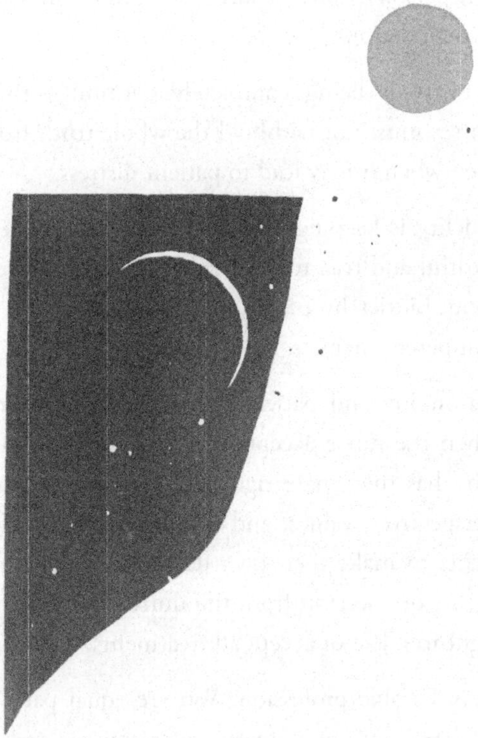

Day 26

A Holy Shift

Change is one of the most consistent qualities of health care. Nursing is in constant motion and constantly morphing. Your profession will continue to throw you curveballs, surprises, and pandemics.

Resilience is the ability to name, face, and transcend difficulty — over and over. This word is carelessly thrown around the nursing profession, but it is actually a practice that must be cultivated.

Think of when you were training for this profession. Remember how overwhelmed you felt when you first drew blood, started an IV, or told a patient they were dying? Over time and with much practice, those skills have come to feel routine. Resilience is like a muscle that requires an ongoing fitness program. Your resilience says, "I got this," even when a part of us says, "No, thank you. This is not what I signed up for. Call me when this is over."

Self-Care Practice

On those days that you are feeling frustrated with a specific aspect of nursing or challenging an unwelcome change, try the following "I have, I am, I can" exercise adapted by MJ Murray Vachon from the International Resilience Project (Grothberg, 1995).

Step 1

Complete the sentence of one or many of the prompts:

Heck no_____.

I am sick of_____.

_____ is not what I signed up for.

_____ is not fair.

I hate _____.

Why do I have to_____?

This is your truth. Write your truth on paper, record it into a voice memo on your phone, or write it in sidewalk chalk. Get it out of your head and into the atmosphere where you can see it once you have dumped it. This is just for you, so misspellings, bad grammar, and curses are fine and encouraged.

For example: When my manager changed my morning start time from 7 a.m. to 4 a.m., mine was: "Heck no, this is not fair. I did not sign up for this. Is this for real? Does she not know how much harder it is to wake up at 3 a.m. than 6 a.m.? Now I have to go to bed at 8 p.m. I hate this. I am not going to do this anymore. I am out of here."

Now, take a few breaths. You have put your truth out there. No one can take your truth from you. Leave it be. Take a break. Go get a drink or go for a walk.

Step 2 (A Bit Later)

Reread or re-listen to your truth.

Is this your whole truth?

Probably not. You probably do not even need to dig deep to answer that, but you may have to put some effort into shifting your mental attitude. This is what builds resilience — transcending the difficult — again and again. Considering your understandable frustrations, ask yourself these questions:

> What support do *I have* that can help me in my work life to manage this change?
>
> What support do *I have* that can help me in my home life?
>
> *Who am I?* What strengths do I have that I can apply to this moment in my life? What feelings, beliefs, and attitudes do I need to connect with to make this holy shift?

For example, I have my lovely co-workers, and they are all agreeable to this change. My manager has made many good decisions in the past — perhaps she sees something I do not see. My husband can drive the kids to school, and I do not like to stay up late anyway. Maybe I can have a conversation with my manager.

What can you *do* that will help resolve your negativity, low self-esteem, frustration, anger, feelings of doom, or overwhelm?

It can be as obvious as changing your sleep schedule or as challenging as talking to your supervisor.

Maybe you need to:

- Up your game in terms of managing your feelings.
- Ask a friend to listen without trying to fix the problem.
- Step into the reality that life is hard, and that does not mean you are messing up. It is the nature of this life we are all living in.

What is your can-do plan?

Resilience is transforming the "holy s**t" moment into a holy shift that reconnects you to your deepest self that is a healer and helper. Commit to your can-do plan, which will facilitate this shift.

My holy shift was having a very long, honest conversation with my boss. She would not relent. The next day I turned in my resignation. She eventually changed the shift times back to a 7 a.m. start time, and I got my job back.

I know many nurses in their 60s and 70s that are bad*ss pivoters — they walk to work during ice storms, they drive 40 miles in the middle of the night to a patient's home, and they learn entirely new computer systems in weeks, all without complaining. The ability to change and shift is in their bones.

This practice can foster a graceful transition for you when you are feeling resistant to or frustrated with any change. Change in health care is ongoing and inevitable.

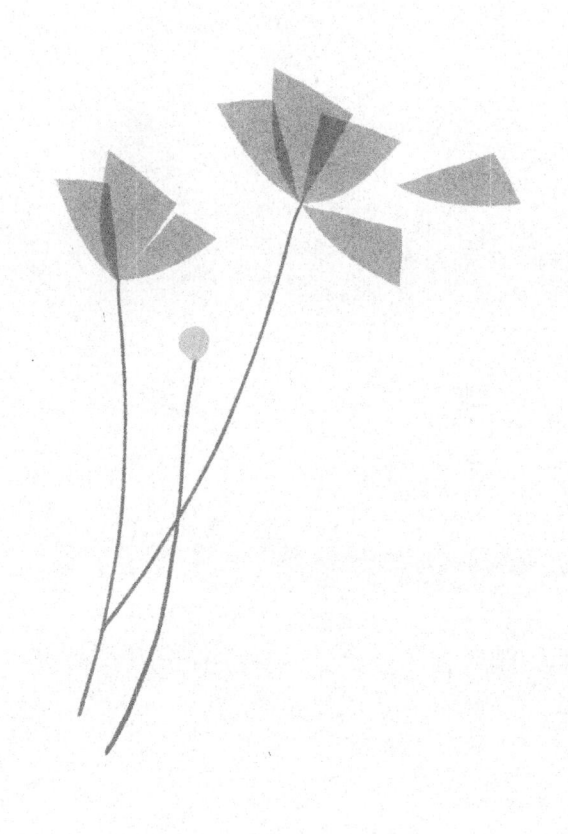

Day 27

Get the Fluffy Tissues

You are trained to do everything possible to keep your patients alive, but sometimes patients die despite your Herculean efforts and expertise.[23]

I took care of a 28-year-old gentleman who was dying from cancer when I was just the same age — his friends and girlfriend were ever-present. I have seen it a few times before, but this young man was lucid, mentally clear, and agitated minutes before he died. He frantically paced around the room as he was actively dying, and only in the last few moments did he acquiesce, lie down in bed with his girlfriend, and die.

It was a dramatic death — too young, too soon, and a startling reminder of my own mortality.

I went home that evening shaken, realizing that death comes

---

[23] One hundred percent of people on this planet will die at some point. Death is as natural as birth, and it should be an essential part of the health care continuum, medical care, and insurance plans.

to all of us, ready or not. It is undiscriminating and ruthless, and this notion turned my world upside down.

Self-Care Practice

As a clinician, you are confronted with your own mortality every day. It is important to consider your own death as you continue to do this work. When you ponder or wrestle with this absolute, you may not take the "medical failures" so personally, or you may be able to empathically support your patient's struggle with their mortality. Or, as in my case, it may encourage you to buy a ticket to Thailand.

Get a box of fluffy tissues and a blanket. Lie down on the floor or your bed. Set your alarm for 30 minutes just in case you fall asleep.

Consider your own mortality. Someday you *will* die. Imagine your death 30 years from now. Just be with it.

What do you want your death to look like? Do you want family members around when you die? What do you want to do before you die? Do you have your own advanced directives written?

Next, imagine your death 10 years from now and ask the same questions. How old will you be? What kind of a life will you have lived? How do you want to leave this earth? Just be with it.

Next, imagine your death one year from now, and ask the same questions above.

This practice may make you feel uncomfortable, unsettled, or angry. Breathe into the discomfort. Take a few more minutes and write about it. Let it settle into your bones a bit. As much control as we think we have (and nurses can be kind of controlling), death is an absolute truth on this earth. We can delay death, avoid death, and keep people alive if the ventilators, feeding tubes, and bypasses allow, but at some point, our lungs will not respond to the usual medical therapies, the burden of tube feeding outweighs the benefit, or new arterial plaques may form. Nobody, except for maybe Elvis, lives forever.

When you contemplate your own human vulnerability, it can soften your nursing heart and perhaps even inspire you to take a vacation.

Day 28

Secondhand Trauma

One night I awoke, startled and sweaty, dreaming about my patient in Room 222 offering me a donut wrapped in saline-soaked gauze. His horrifying dressing change from the previous shift immediately came flashing back. Now I was wide awake at 3 a.m. replaying his story and dressing change in my head. I was not going back to sleep, and I probably would not be able to eat a donut for a while either.

Some days certain patients, their story, or their body parts will lodge into our memories and may be difficult to release. You cannot unsee or un-experience difficult events, and sometimes they seep into your psyche. This is called *secondhand trauma*. Laura van Dernoot Lipsky, founder of The Trauma Steward Institute, explains that first responders can experience this condition when they hear about a traumatic event or see the physical signs of the traumatic event. Secondhand trauma can manifest in various ways including diminished creativity, chronic exhaustion, and hopelessness.

When I heard the term *secondhand trauma* after I had been a nurse for 20 years, I was angry.[24] Why is this not a discussion in our nursing culture? Should we not be proactive in healing the healer? We should have therapists on-site and 30-minute timeouts after we are thrown off our game by any death, brutal resuscitation, or even an explosive poop. But until that happens, we simply must take this manner into our own hands and aim to move through these events with some grace.

Self-Care Practice

Research shows you must regularly work through how the intense events that you experience at work affect you (Vachon, 2020; Figley, 2002). According to van Dernoot Lipsky, diet, exercise, restorative sleep, creative expression, time spent in nature, or therapy can help to heal secondhand trauma (The Trauma Stewardship Institute Home, 2018).

For today's practice, you will focus on creative expression. For all of you nurses who recoiled from that sentence, an inability to embrace creative expression is one of the effects of secondhand trauma. So, take a breath, and please, just try this.

Grab a piece of blank paper and some colored markers or a colored pen. To get technical and precise, you can use a ruler and a compass, but the goal is not perfection. Find a table in

---

[24] Of course, another long phone call with my cousin MJ led me to this insight. I told her about how I was feeling after I experienced a terrible death, and she said, "Oh yeah, that's secondhand trauma." I felt angry but also felt the relief of giving my feelings a name.

your home, turn on some music, and take a minute to settle in. You are going to create a mandala. Place a dot in the center of your blank page. Draw a circle around this dot — it can be one-fourth an inch wide or more. Then continue to draw concentric circles around this circle using the same center point. Draw as many circles as you like — you may have up to 10 circles within one circle.

Next, draw a pattern within each circle. The patterns available for you to use are unlimited — they can be lines, flower petal shapes, triangles, circles, or squares. Use the words *repetition*, *symmetry*, and *flow* to guide you. If you want, you can color within your designs and patterns, paying attention to symmetry.

The mandala is a spiritual symbol rooted in Buddhism and Hinduism that dates to the fifth century, though the symbol can be found in many other cultural traditions. Creating mandalas were a form of meditation and prayer. Mandalas were introduced as a therapeutic intervention by psychoanalyst Carl Jung. The Jungian tradition uses mandalas as a tool "for self-awareness, conflict resolution, and as a basis for various other art psychotherapeutic techniques in a variety of situations" (Slegelis, 1987, p. 301).

Move through this practice with patience, openness, and curiosity. Notice any words, thoughts, or images that come to mind. With this exercise, make sure to laugh a bit, play a bit, and pay attention to any personal insights or reflections that arise while drawing. You may want to write about what came up during the practice after completing your mandala.

Day 29

A Soft Front and a Strong Back

About a year into my hospice work, I was depressed and grumpy — apparently this is common.[25] I wanted to continue this work and to show up for my patients and their suffering without the accompanying depression. I tried a few things to protect myself; I felt a little less, I detached myself, and I tried to envision a bubble around me that walled me off from my patients' emotions.

I tried these practices for a week. The technique of separating myself and emotionally disengaging actually had a more disturbing effect on me. I started to like my job a little less, and I cared a little less about my patients. I felt cut off and disconnected from the beauty of the work.

---

25 Bernice Harper discovered five stages one experiences when working with dying patients. Depression is Stage 3. The five stages, in order, are 1) intellectualization, 2) emotional survival, 3) depression, 4) emotional arrival, 5) deep compassion (Harper, 1977/1994).

I wanted more reciprocity. I wanted my patients to know that I truly cared about them without the accompanying depression.

On a retreat, Joan Halifax, a Buddhist teacher and Zen priest, taught me about the soft front/strong back approach to caring for the dying. Your soft front is your compassion for your patients that allows you to consider your patients' circumstances with an open heart, not a broken heart (Halifax et al., 2007).

The strong back is your equanimity, the centeredness that comes from an inner wisdom and the truth that some things are fixable while some are not. Many patients will suffer, and you cannot take away their suffering, but you can bear witness to their suffering.

Halifax's approach matches what the science of compassion research has found, specifically that compassion is being moved by the suffering to do whatever you can for another person knowing that you do not have complete control over the outcome; what counts is that you do your best (Vachon, 2020). Compassion allows you to resonate with the joy or suffering of another but simultaneously understand that these are not your personal emotions (Singer & Klimecki, 2014).

Self-Care Practice

Find a comfortable seat. Look at the following phrases from Halifax's book, "Being With Dying" (Halifax et al., 2007, pp. 74–75). Slowly, intentionally, with each breath, say each phrase.

May the power of loving kindness sustain me.

May you be happy and free of pain.

May all those who suffer be free of pain.

May I offer my care and presence unconditionally, knowing it may be met by gratitude, indifference, anger, or anguish.

May I offer love knowing that I cannot control the course of life, suffering, or death.

May I remain in peace and let go of expectations.

I care about your pain and suffering. May I be present for it.

I will care for you, and I cannot take away your suffering.

May I accept things as they are.

I wish you happiness and peace. I cannot make your choices for you.

May I see my limits compassionately just as I view the suffering of others.

May I and all beings live and die in ease.

You may want to circle or copy to a notebook the ones that resonate for you so you can come back to them when you need to hold yourself with a soft front and a strong back.

A nurse's mission is to heal the patient — their wounds and their diseases. As you continue to walk this profession, you realize that sometimes the chemo treatment fails, infections recur, or the patient's pain is intractable. But if we can show up for our shift with compassion and the accompanying equanimity, we can foster our patient's healing in some way. It may not be healing of the body, but your presence could soften their fear, prevent their feelings of isolation, and in the end, may help heal their spirit, which is sometimes, oftentimes, just as important as healing their body.

Day 30

Too Much Fight or Flight

If you work in health care, you are constantly responding to literal crises: sudden chest pain, altered mental status, a decrease in urine output, or blood pressure tanking. You must spring into action and fix these malfunctioning body parts — quickly. When people are in the hospital, patients and family members often arrive in crisis. Flights for other family members have not been booked, care has not been arranged, and priests have not been summoned. You are literally working in the middle of a crisis inside of a crisis inside of a crisis.

Our fight-or-flight response is what allows us to spring and respond to a crisis. When it happens over and over again, we spring, then we spring, and then we spring again. Then you are thrown a death, an extra shift, and maybe a pandemic, and your circuits blow. When you are under constant stress, you cannot access higher-order thinking. Often, nurses become physically and mentally depleted.

Self-Care Practice

Yes, you can respond to multiple crises again and again and again, but you must balance that with healing, again and again and again. I would love for this book to contain a month-long trip to Hawaii, a massage, and a mai tai for every nurse who reads it. That can sometimes be necessary and well-deserved for those dealing with chronic stress, but alas, reality.

For our final day together, I ask you to tap into that compassion you freely offer to your patients and direct it toward yourself. Take a slow walk for a half-hour and contemplate the last 29 days. You can do the next exercise lying down if you are simply too d**n tired.

Walk thoughtfully while breathing intentionally. Slower and fewer steps are encouraged. Pay attention to the sights and sounds as you consider your bad*ss nursing self: the good that you do, your commitment to others' health and well-being, your ethical precepts that drive your practice and possibly your life, your compassion for your patients, your trust in your co-workers, your clinical competence, your strength, your brilliance, and your no-BS attitude.

Nurses are a rare breed. You have to be kind and gentle with your beautiful self. Compassion science research notes that human beings are healthiest when they become comfortable expressing compassion to others, can accept compassion from others, and are able to be compassionate toward themselves (Gilbert, 2014). You must take the time to nurture, to nourish, and to heal yourself.

Conclusion

A Love Letter to Nurses

As I wrote this little guidebook, it became clear that in addition to supporting nurses, this book is a celebration of nurses. I am blown away by all that you do.

You run, you sprint, you lift, you hoist, you squat, you inject, and you lunge.

You handle poop, vomit, phlegm, sputum, discharge, urine, blood, and bodily fluids of all different colors, consistencies, and volumes. And you can describe them, in great detail.

You coo, you soothe, you hold, you love, you stroke, you reassure, and you cherish.

You start IVs, hang blood, insert catheters and rectal tubes, administer medications, reattach colostomies, and master new computer programs in real time.

You arrive early and work late. You work extra shifts, and you get flexed without pay. You work in the most inclement weather — there are no snow days for nurses.

You are present for life's celebrations: births, remissions, cures, and recovery.

You bear witness to profound suffering: falls, motor vehicle accidents, burns, recurrences, and death.

You are in close proximity to the harsh realities of life: addiction, trauma, suicide, homelessness, isolation, mental illness, and inadequate everything.

You educate families in crisis, you explain to the pacing son, you reassure the patient's daughter, and you mentor the baby doctors.

You have a soft heart and a no-BS attitude, a brilliant mind with a get-er-done spirit. You are a truth seeker and truth teller, powerful advocate and quiet bystander, scientist and mystic, god, and goddess, angel and warrior.

And when a pandemic hits, you work in chaotic conditions, with protocols, regulations, rules, and walls changing every day. You pivot, you work with inadequate safety supplies, and literally risk your lives for the good of the community.

You do it all.

You are everything wrapped up into one perfect human package.

This little guidebook is written to support you as you continue the beautiful work of nursing for as long as you want to do it. I see you, and I celebrate you. I hope this guidebook has given you 30 ways to nurture, honor, and celebrate yourself in the difficult work that you do.

Written with great love and admiration,

Beth

Bibliography

Burke, A. (2021, February 15). Ethical practice: NCLEX RN. Registered Nursing. https://www.registered-nursing.org/nclex/ethical-practice/

Dagar, C., Pandey, A., & Navare, A. (2020). How yoga-based practices build altruistic behavior? Examining the role of subjective vitality, self-transcendence, and psychological capital. *Journal of Business Ethics*, 1–16.

Dillard, J. P., Yang, C., & Li, R. (2018, July). *Self-regulation of emotional responses to Zika: Spiral of fear.* Plos One. https://journals.plos.org/plosone/article?id=10.1371/journal.pone.0199828

Emmons, E. R., & Mishra, A. (2011). Why gratitude enhances well-being: What we know, what we need to know. In K. M. Sheldon, T. B. Kashdan, & M. F. Steger (Eds.), *Designing positive psychology: Taking stock and moving forward* (pp. 248–262). Oxford University Press.

Figley, C. R. (2002). *Treating compassion fatigue*. Brunner-Routledge.

Gilbert, P. (2014). The origins and nature of compassion focused therapy. *British Journal of Clinical Psychology*, 53(1), 6–41.

Goetz, J. L., Keltner, D., & Simon-Thomas, E. (2010). Compassion: An evolutionary analysis and empirical review. *Psychological Bulletin*, 136(3), 351–374.

Gotter, A., & Weatherspoon, D. (2020, June 17). *Box breathing*. Healthline. https://www.healthline.com/health/box-breathing

Grothberg, E. (1995). A guide to promoting resilience in children: Strengthening the human spirit. (Early Childhood Development: Practice and Reflections Series, Number 8). International Resilience Project, 1–43.

Halifax, J., Dossey, B. M., & Rushton, C. H. (2007). *Being with dying: Compassionate end-of-life-care training guide*. Pranja Mountain Publishers.

Harper, B. C. (1994). *Death: The coping mechanism of the health professional*. Swinger Associates. (Original work published 1977)

Invaluable. (2018, December 19). What is a mandala? History, symbolism, and uses. https://www.invaluable.com/blog/what-is-a-mandala/

Kent, T. L. (2014). *Wild creative igniting your passion and potential in work, home, and life*. Atria Paperback.

Loehr, J., & Schwartz, T. (2003). *The power of full engagement: Managing energy, not time is the key to high performance and personal renewal*. Free Press.

Malchiodi, C. (2010, March 17). *Cool art therapy inter-*

vention #6: Mandala drawing. Psychology Today. https://www.psychologytoday.com/us/blog/arts-and-health/201003/cool-art-therapy-intervention-6-mandala-drawing

Porges, S. W. (2017). Vagal pathways: Portals to compassion. In E. M. Seppälä, E. Simon-Thomas, S. L. Brown, M. C. Worline, C. D. Cameron, & J. R. Doty (Eds.), *The Oxford handbook of compassion science* (pp. 189–202). Oxford University Press.

Porges, Stephen W. *Polyvagal Safety: Attachment, Communication, Safety, Self-Regulation* (p. 70). New York: W. W. Norton & Company 2021.

Salzberg, S. (2002). *Loving-kindness: The revolutionary art of happiness.* Shambhala.

Seppälä, E., Bradley, C., & Goldstein, M. (2020, September 9). Research: Why breathing is so effective at reducing stress. Harvard Business Review. https://hbr.org/2020/09/research-why-breathing-is-so-effective-at-reducing-stress

Siegel, D. J. (2015). *Brainstorm: The power and purpose of the teenage brain.* TarcherPerigee.

Singer, T., & Klimecki, O. (2014). Empathy and compassion. *Current Biology, 24*(18), R875–R878.

Slegelis, M. H. (1987). A study of Jung's mandala and its relationship to art psychotherapy. *The Arts in Psychotherapy, 14*(4), 301–311. https://doi.org/10.1016/0197-4556(87)90018-9

The Trauma Stewardship Institute. (2018). Laura van dernoot lipsky. https://traumastewardship.com/laura-van-dernoot-lipsky/

Vachon, D. O. (2020). *How doctors care: The science of compassionate and balanced caring in medicine.* Cognella Press.

Watson, J. (2008). *Nursing, the philosophy and science of caring.* The University Press of Colorado.

Watson, J. (2021). *10 caritas processes.* Watson Caring Science Institute. https://www.watsoncaringscience.org/jean-bio/caring-science-theory/10-caritas-processes/

Weng, H. Y., Schuyler, B., & Da, R. J. (2017). The impact of compassion meditation training on the brain and prosocial behavior. In E. M. Seppälä, E. Simon-Thomas, S. L. Brown, M. C. Worline, C. D. Cameron, & J. R. Doty (Eds.), *Oxford Handbook of Compassion Science,* 133-146.

Zaccaro, A., Piarulli, A., Laurino, M., Garbella, E., Menicucci, D., Neri, B., & Gemignani, A. (2018, September 7). How breath-control can change your life: A systematic review on psycho-physiological correlates of slow breathing. *Frontiers in Human Neuroscience, 12*(353).

Acknowledgements

I wrote this book in the spirit of constant gratitude and humility. This book would not exist if it were not for MJ Murray Vachon LCSW, LMFT, Dominic Vachon MDiv, PhD, and Colleen Sweeney RN, BS, CSP. They are collaborators, researchers, and thought provokers for this book. It is essentially our book. I am also grateful for my brilliant, kind, and thoughtful editor, Mira Petrillo, who continues to give me the courage to write. She collaborated with me throughout the entire project, helped me form and shape the book, and then helped give birth to the book baby. She is my book doula. Lastly, I always want to acknowledge my husband, Kevin. He does not know it, but he is my Yoda, my constant cheerleader who gives me ongoing courage with his just-do-it-and-follow-your-heart-your-soul-your-passions attitude — regardless of the outcome.

Made in the USA
Las Vegas, NV
13 January 2025